March 29, 2010
Dear Rita,
May this book
truly bless you!
H.C

Sex and Marriage: Myths Uncovered

Sex and Marriage: Myths Uncovered

Dr. Cynthia L. McGill

VANTAGE PRESS
New York

The letters contained herein are fictitious. Any similarity between the names and characters in this book and any real persons, living or dead, is purely coincidental.

FIRST EDITION

All rights reserved, including the right of reproduction in whole or in part in any form.

Copyright © 2009 by Dr. Cynthia L. McGill

Published by Vantage Press, Inc.
419 Park Ave. South, New York, NY 10016

Manufactured in the United States of America
ISBN: 978-0-533-16164-5

Library of Congress Catalog Card No.: 2008910825

0 9 8 7 6 5 4 3 2 1

To the six loves of my life:
My Lord and Saviour, Jesus Christ
My supporter, best friend, lover and husband, Reginald
My cheerleader and role model, my mom, Doris Tarpley
My girls, Maia, Adrienne and Gabby who are my heart

Have nothing to do with godless myths and old wives' tales; rather, train yourself to be godly. For physical training is of some value, but godliness has value for all things, holding promise for both the present life and the life to come.

—I Timothy 4:7–8 (NIV)

Contents

Introduction	1
Myth #1: Love Is All We Need	7
Myth #2: Marriage Will Complete Me	20
Myth #3: I Can Change Him!	31
Myth #4: No More Single Girlfriends for Me . . . I's Married Now!	41
Myth #5: It's Not My Job to Build Him Up!	51
Myth #6: He Should Be More Like Me!	66
Myth #7: "Submission" Is Optional for a Good Marriage	78
Myth #8: We Will Never Argue	88
Myth #9: Love No Longer Lives Here	99
Myth #10: Sex Is Love	110

Sex and Marriage: Myths Uncovered

Introduction

Dissatisfaction. Displeasure. Distress. Discontent. Disenchantment. Disillusionment. These are sure to come for women who are looking for the Cinderella-like happily-ever-after fairy-tale marriage. Do you recall or have you watched *The Cosby Show, Ozzie and Harriet, Little House on the Prairie, I Love Lucy, The Honeymooners, The Donna Reed Show, Cinderella,* and the comic strips *Blondie,* and *Hi & Lois*? These marriages didn't seem to have any real problems.

When I got married over thirty-six years ago, little did I realize how many myths I held about marriage. For example, I thought, "my husband should be more like me," "submission to my husband is not necessary to make a good marriage," and more. If you had asked me where I got those beliefs, I could not tell you. Perhaps it was these television shows, comic strips, magazines and movies.

What myths do you hold about marriage? Are you ready to have some marriage myths exposed for what they really are—fiction, false images and just plain unreal? Good, thriving, nurturing marriages are not grown in test tubes nor in fairy tales but in a relationship with a man and woman (with all their faults) making a commitment to consistently work on loving and serving one another as Christ loves and serves His church.

The *Women's Study Bible* states:

Marriage is a three-fold miracle.
1. **A Biological Miracle** because two people are actually be-

coming one flesh. You begin to think alike. You begin to finish your spouse's sentences.
2. **A Social Miracle** because his family and your family are actually grafted together. His family is now your family and vice versa.
3. **A Spiritual Miracle** because the marriage relationship is meant to be equivalent to the union between God and his bride, the church.

We must understand that marriage is the highest of all human commitments. There is absolutely no room for selfishness. Your goal is to love your spouse as an illustration of your love for the Lord.

My husband and I have had to recommit to one another and to our marriage many times. Have we felt like giving up? Absolutely! Are we going to give up? No! While I absolutely adore my husband and he is still the only man who makes my heart do flips, and makes my face light up every time I see him, we have seen our share of hardships, challenges, financial lows, inexplicable joys, and romantic passion. However, we had to commit to God and to each other for life. We also had to expose the marital myths we held as truths and become less self-centered, make God the center of our marriage, and unload some heavy personal baggage. Then, and only then, did we truly start loving each other as God ordained.

My husband and I have counseled hundreds of couples during our twenty-five-year ministry—in our church as well as in marriage retreats. We learned that many false beliefs were hindering couples from having a fulfilled, happy marriage. I also held focus groups with married ladies in my church. They were open and forthcoming with myths they believed. Those discussions as well as my experiences as a married woman and a Pastor have influenced the contents of this book.

And no one puts a piece of cloth that has not been shrunk on an old garment, for such a patch tears away from the garment and a

> *worse rent (tear) is made. Neither is new wine put in old wineskins; for if it is, the skins burst and are torn in pieces, and the wine is spilled and the skins are ruined. But new wine is put into fresh wineskins, and so both are preserved.*
> —Matthew 9:16–17 AMP

Just as Jesus did not come to "patch up" the old holier-than-thou system of Judaism with its sets of laws and customs, I did not come to boost, bolster or support the myths of marriage that could cause you years of hurt. My resolve for writing this book is to bring genuineness, reality and truth into the thoughts of twenty-first-century women who are single and waiting for a companion, divorced and trusting God for another marriage, as well as women who are married and want "new wine" in their fresh marriage wineskin.

When you become like "new wine" in "new wine skin" you will enjoy a rewarding life journey with your spouse. Marriage simply cannot work if you are trying to have a "new you" co-exist with your old, flawed behaviors and ideologies. This permanent shift in attitude will prevent you from encountering frustrations that can lead to behaviors that can sabotage your marriage. You will be free to love your husband, as described in I Corinthians 13, and willing to submit to him as described in the fifth chapter of Ephesians.

> *Wives, be subject [be submissive and adapt yourselves] to your own husbands as [a service] to the Lord . . . As the church is subject to Christ, so let wives also be subject in everything to their husbands . . . However, let each man of you [without exception] love his wife as [being in a sense] his very own self; and let the wife see that she respects and reverences her husband [that she notices him, regards him, honors him, prefers him, venerates, and esteems him; and that she defers to him, praises him, and loves and admires him exceedingly].*
> —Ephesians 5:22, 24, 33 AMP

In this passage of scripture we are told what is required to have healthy and fulfilling relationships with our spouses. Our ultimate goal as women, either married or wanting to be married, is to put aside selfish behaviors and desires that hamper our ability to have successful marriages. We must prepare ourselves to become partner-focused rather than self-focused. The scripture in Matthew metaphorically tells us that we have to abandon our old system of thinking that may have produced negative ways of functioning in our marriages. Not only are we to approach marriage with a new attitude and outlook, but there should also be tangible evidence that we have really worked on ourselves.

In order to alert more women to marital myths and expose the devil for who he is (a fraud, robber of joy and contract killer of marriages), I determined to put pen to paper and expose the darkness that surrounds ten myths that can prevent women from having a genuine loving marriage.

Who should read this book? Those women who have been married for twenty years or less. For you, this book will shed light into some dark places where some of these myths are stored. For those women who are single. I say to you, expose those myths now! Do not wait!

I believe a marriage needs love, encouragement, patience, communication, reasonable expectations, attention, cultivation, and a sense of humor to survive and thrive. Marriage is not for the fainthearted. It is not for wimps. You must have a "stick to it" mentality when it comes to marriage. Otherwise you will desire a divorce at the first sign of discomfort. Marriage requires you to share such things as your bed, your bank account, household chores, how you plan to raise your children, where you are going and what time you will be home, etc. If you do not like including another person in almost all of your decisions, if you do not like doing things that you would rather not do, if you do not like consulting with someone else regarding how you are going to spend your money, if you do not like being accountable to your spouse in virtually every way—please, please do not get married! Marriage is not for selfish people.

Even after going through months of premarital counseling, we seem to get amnesia after we get married. Often times, we go back to our old selfish behaviors. It's almost as if we say, "Well I have him now, so I can go back to being that old person who wants things entirely my way." For example, we may decide that we don't want to help pay the bills. We use phrases like "this is my money." In blended families, we restrict our spouse from being a part of the disciplinary process with our children. We want marriage to be convenient and to love our spouses only as long as they are doing what we want them to do. God will constantly challenge us to abandon this selfish and destructive way of thinking. His desire is for us to be flexible for the good of the relationship and to love each other in God's terms as described in I Corinthians 13:4–7.

As we pursue Christ the Lord throughout these pages, get geared up for fresh ways to live, new-found ways to look at your husband, and new ways to function. So, let's roll up our sleeves, grab a bottle of water or a cup of coffee and a pen and get started!

Lay Bare Your Soul . . . Expose yourself to the truth!
Behold, You desire truth in the inner being; make me therefore to know
wisdom in my inmost heart.
—Psalms 51:6

What are some of your marriage myths?

_____
_____
_____
_____

Why do you think there is often discomfort in the cleaving (adhering) process of marriage? How can you or how did you prepare to be more "partner-focused" rather than "self-focused"?

_____
_____
_____
_____

In your own words what does I Corinthians 13:4–7 mean to you? Contrast that with infatuation.

_____
_____
_____
_____

Myth #1: Love Is All We Need

*There's nothing you can do that can't be done.
Nothing you can sing that can't be sung.
Nothing you can say but you can learn how to play the game.
It's easy.*
"Love Is All You Need," The Beatles

One of the most popular songs in the 1960s was "Love Is All You Need" by The Beatles. This song tries to imitate a romantic love between a male and female from the Greek word **eros**. Men and women of today are still trying to satisfy emptiness in their spirit, appealing for something genuine and sincere. A lot of men and women get married with the idea that love will fulfill and satisfy them. Even more men and women have sex outside of marriage for the same purpose but in its place get back lust in all the inappropriate ways.

The truth of the matter was (let's just tell the truth now ladies): "Lust is all I need." When I first laid eyes on Reginald Allen McGill, my heart did flips, my palms started sweating and my knees almost buckled. I was having a chemical reaction to this very nice, handsome, charming man. For both of us, it was "love" at first sight. However, in reality, it was actually "lust" at first sight. Neither one of us had the slightest idea of how to love each other as God ordained.

A lasting marriage cannot be rooted in infatuation. Infatuation by definition means to be "completely carried away by unreasoning passion and attraction." Although this phase of marriage is extremely emotion-charged, this is not real love. During this stage, you are giggly, hanging on to every word that your spouse speaks and are completely enamored with his intellect, wisdom, and knowledge. All of his positive attributes are magnified. This temporary period of your relationship is based on romantic feelings, physical attraction, and good old-fashioned lust. For the first few years (or months) this is exactly how it should be. However, as with anything rooted exclusively in emotion, this period of marriage does not and should not last.

Although we know before marriage that no one is perfect, our attitude, when our spouse disagrees with us or says something that we consider to be unacceptable, begins to change with time. The excitement of the early relationship diminishes, and the result is that we no longer feel happy. Each time we feel disappointed, each time that our feelings get hurt, an emotional brick is formed, and before you know it you have created a whole wall of resentment.

That wall of resentment starts as a small layer of bricks called disappointment, and then comes a layer of anger, followed by layers of resentment and bitterness. Before you know it, you are not talking to your husband (not any real, meaningful communication anyway) and you both soon become just housemates.

Love in marriage is about meeting the marital (not spiritual) needs of your spouse. After more than thirty-six years of marriage and countless arguments, a myriad of "I'm sorry" statements, teary-eyed prayers, and romantic "I love you" declarations, I can honestly say I did not start to understand that meeting my husband's marital needs *is* love until about year fifteen of our marriage.

We got married six months after I graduated from college. I was starry-eyed and quite naïve about most things. Reginald, already four years out of college, thought he was ready for a commitment as well. Neither one of us knew how to meet each other's marital needs (well, not all of them—SMILES!). Both of us were selfish and self-centered. I wanted everything "my way" and he wanted everything "his way"; except, he was less vocal. I let him know exactly how I felt—at all times. When I was upset, angry, depressed, sad or happy, he knew it. However, I never quite knew how he truly felt because he would not (actually at that time, he could not) share his feelings with me.

Most men have a harder time expressing their true feelings. Often, they do not even know what their true feelings are especially if they are trying to be a "good" husband without even knowing what a "good" husband is truly. Only a husband who strives to meet his spouse's marital needs through constant, open and sincere communication, with the help of God, can even begin to have a fulfilling marriage.

I soon learned men's and women's marital needs are quite different. Couples often fail to meet each other's marital needs.

> Ignorance contributes to this failure because men and women have great difficulty understanding and appreciating the value of each other's needs. Men tend to try to meet needs that they would value and women do the same. The problem is that the needs of men and women are often very different and we waste effort trying to meet the wrong needs.
> —Willard F. Harley Jr., *His Needs, Her Needs: Building an Affair-Proof Marriage.* Baker Book House Company, Grand Rapids, MI., 2001, pg. 15.

Marital needs include laying aside your selfish needs for your spouse's. For example, listening attentively even when you do not feel like it; taking the kids out of the house for most of the day so your spouse can have a day "off"; supporting your spouse when he/she wants to go back to school; encouraging your spouse to be the best person he/she can be; saying "I'm sorry" even though you do not think it's your fault, etc.

However, what happens when your husband will not meet your marital needs? Let us dissect this question into three parts:

- Some husbands want to meet their wives' marital needs but do not know how, but want to learn.
- Some husbands do not know how but do not want to learn.
- There are those men who do not know how but do not know they don't know.

Let us deal with each group of men separately. If your husband does not know how, but wants to learn, then you are already well on your way to oneness. Attend as many Christian Married Couples retreats as you both can together. Have a steady diet of Christian marital books and study guides. Discuss them together. Pray together. Go to counseling together. Forgive each other. Encourage each other. Ask your spouse: What can I do to be a better wife to you? What needs do you have that I can meet? Listen carefully. Then, restate what you have heard. Get a true understanding of what your husband is asking of you. Can you meet those needs? Do you need to ask him to compromise? For example, if he wants you to cook five times a week but you truly feel you can only cook three times a week consistently, tell him. Then, ask him if he will be happy with that compromise. Then, you both need to discuss how you will eat the other four days of the week. Once you have discussed how you can best meet his needs and you have settled on answers that you are both comfortable with, then it is his turn to ask you: What can I do to be a better husband? What needs of yours can I meet?

What happens if your husband does not know how to meet your marital needs but does not want to learn? My sister, you must pray and ask God for a miracle in your marriage. Only the miracle working power of the Holy Spirit can convict your husband, prick his heart, and awake him to desire to learn to meet your needs. You must realize that you cannot change your husband. All the nagging and arguing in the world will not change your husband.

Have you tried to deal with one need at a time? Stop trying to confront him with five needs at a time. For example, if you want him to communicate more openly and effectively with you, have you asked him? Have you approached him, after prayer, and asked him can you both go for walks one evening a week together? Do not say, so we can talk; just say a walk. The first time you go for a walk, do not say a word, unless he does. Wait until the Lord tells you to talk and ask the Lord what you should say. If you have ever "shut him down" in the past, then you will have to build his trust in your ability not to be judgmental when he does share what is on his heart. The Lord may lead you two to talk about the neighboring lawns, the dogs barking (in other words, trivial stuff). You both may laugh at something together or even may start holding hands. Just let the Lord orchestrate what happens on these walks; you stay out of God's way! There is a lot of "communication" that can take place in silence. Allow yourself just to enjoy his company and vice versa without nagging, judging or even begging for something that rightfully he should be willing to give you. You must allow the Holy Spirit to do all the work. Eventually, your husband will start talking and you must learn to listen without judgment or castigation or interruptions, if you want him to continue to be open with you. As you see the Lord working on your communication issue, you will have more faith to believe God can work on the other issues in your marriage.

Then, there is the final group of husbands who do not know how to meet your needs but do not even know they don't meet your needs. Pray and ask God which Christian couple in your church would be a good role model for you and your husband. Suggest to your husband that you would like to invite them over for dinner. Start spending time with that couple so that you both can model positive marital behavior. Pray to God to even set up the conversations so that the other couple's husband and wife can share some insight that would be helpful to your marriage. Do not plan it; your husband will see right through the "insight." Let God orchestrate the interaction.

As you can see, I talk a lot about praying. My sister, prayer is the key to unlocking your husband's heart.

Spiritual needs, on the other hand, can only be fulfilled by God. No human, not even your spouse, can fill the void in your deep inner being. No human can make you happy nor make you feel whole and complete. If we put the entire burden on another human being to make us happy, what responsibility do we have to ourselves?

The Beatles were right to some extent if you look at the words of the song from a special view. All you need *is* love; the God kind of love, flowing from our heavenly Father, satisfying our heart with His presence. It is in His presence that we discover completeness.

> I am the vine; you are the branches. Whoever lives in Me and I in Him bears much [abundant] fruit. However, apart from Me [cut off from vital union with Me] you can do nothing.
> —John 15:5 (AMP)

Jesus reveals that the only way to live a happy life is to stay near Him, like a branch attached to the vine. He understands that only His love can really fulfill us and bring about harmony and joyfulness. His love fortifies our lives for a victorious marriage. I was constantly looking for my husband to make me happy. When in actuality, I finally had to look to Jesus for inner joy and peace.

Before saying "I do," please, please, please seek God to meet your spiritual needs. (For further discussion on this subject, I would encourage you to read my book, *Journey to Wholeness*.) If you seek out God before you are even married, there will be a clear distinction in your marriage because the Holy Spirit will reveal God's power of love. If you are already married, it is time to step out into your marriage in a brand new and loving way.

Here are several ways you can step out into your marriage in a new and loving manner! First, you and your husband need a vision for your marriage. "Where there is no vision, the people perish," (Proverbs 29:18a) and that includes your marriage. You need love and a clear vision or plan for your marriage.

Start by sitting down together and listing the components of your marriage: finances, spirituality, sexual needs, household needs, raising and caring for children, etc. I know it may sound overwhelming but just deal with one category at a time. For example, in the area of finances, do you and your husband want to be out of debt in five years? What steps will you both have to take to accomplish this deed? Do you need to seek a debt reduction counselor for guidance? Go through each category and ask each other pertinent questions. Write down the questions then write down the decisions you both make together.

Second, ask yourself, am I meeting my husband's marital needs? Do I even know what his needs are in our marriage? Have I even asked him? We often do things for our husband that we like rather than what he actually likes. I found myself giving cards to my husband with cute little love notes. He certainly enjoys my cards but he would much rather I fix him a meal or bring him a sweet treat from the bakery or remind him to take something very important on a trip that he would have otherwise forgotten.

Ask your husband what he specifically needs from you as his wife. He may say: "I need you to support me more; cook more; or, I need more sex from you." Whatever his marital needs are, you must be willing to discuss how you can best meet them.

Marriage is a complex relationship; the most intricate of all relationships. Unfortunately, most of us do not realize what we are getting into when we say, "I do." There were no pre-marital classes when my husband and I were engaged over thirty-six years ago. The most we were offered was a half-hour (actually, twenty minutes) session with the minister who was going to officiate our wedding.

Deciding on a mate is one of the most critical decisions we make in our natural life. It is a phase in life that is not to be taken casually. If you are not married yet, you should prudently think about the important decision of choosing a mate. Singles, if you are reading this book, I want to commend you. I cannot encourage you enough to not let lust take you over. Stop and ask yourself vital, and often, life-saving questions such as: are his little idiosyncrasies cute or are they going to impede my spiritual growth, damage my self-esteem, or hurt me physically? If the man you are seriously dating is not as serious about the Lord as you are or not even saved, you may be jeopardizing your own spiritual walk with God.

The Bible says in II Corinthians 6:14:

> *Do not be unequally yoked with unbelievers [do not make mismated alliances with them or come under a different yoke with them, inconsistent with your faith]. For what partnership has right living and right standing with God with iniquity and lawlessness? Or how can light have fellowship with darkness?*
>
> —(AMP)

If your fiancé belittles you, disrespects you or your ideas, does not want you to return or finish school, please do not think this is so cute. Ask someone you trust and respect how they perceive the way he talks to you and treats you. Usually, we do not recognize the early signs when someone is damaging our self-esteem, especially if we believe we are "in love." However, someone else can see things a lot clearer and will tell you the truth, if you will only ask. Then, LISTEN!

A happy, strong, lifelong relationship is the aspiration of every married person. It is the plan of God that the marriage experience be an exquisite gift to us.

> Now the Lord God said, It is not good [sufficient, satisfactory] that the man should be alone; I will make him a help meet [suitable, adapted, complementary] for him. And out of the ground the Lord God formed every [wild] beast and living creature of the field and

> every bird of the air and brought them to Adam to see what he would call them; and whatever Adam called every living creature, that was its name. And Adam gave names to all the livestock and to the birds of the air and to every [wild] beast of the field; but for Adam there was not found a help meet [suitable, adapted, complementary] for him. And the Lord God caused a deep sleep to fall upon Adam; and while he slept, He took one of his ribs or a part of his side and closed up the [place with] flesh. And the rib or part of his side which the Lord God had taken from the man He built up and made into a woman, and He brought her to the man. Then Adam said, This [creature] is now bone of my bones and flesh of my flesh; she shall be called Woman, because she was taken out of a man. Therefore a man shall leave his father and his mother and shall become united and cleave to his wife, and they shall become one flesh.
> —Genesis 2:18–24 (AMP)

To be quite honest with you, the whole cleaving concept scared me speechless! Whenever I read that scripture in Bible Study or I heard it recited at weddings, my throat would tighten and my body would shudder. I would think: "What in the world does 'cleave' mean? How does it apply to me?"

Initially I thought "cleave"—becoming one flesh—meant I would have to lose my own identity. Go ahead and confess; you thought the same thing, didn't you? Let us examine the last two verses closely:

> Then Adam said, This [creature] is now bone of my bones and flesh of my flesh; she shall be called Woman, because she was taken out of a man. Therefore a man shall leave his father and his mother and shall become united and cleave to his wife, and they shall become one flesh.
> —Genesis 2:23–24 (AMP)

The 23rd verse clearly reminds ladies just how much God loves us. <u>God took us out of the man</u>. We are an integral, essential, vital part of our husbands. Ladies, we must embrace this truth; we must celebrate this truth; we must understand and live this truth which is the direct Word of God.

The 24th verse lets us know that our husbands, once married, must leave his parents (i.e. "leave" their home and "leave" their parental control) and become united—one flesh—with his wife. I can hear single women asking: "But what about me?" Until you are married, God is your direct covering. After marriage, God is the head of the husband and your husband becomes your direct covering. In Ephesians 5:22–23(AMP) it reads:

> *Wives, be subject [be submissive and adapt yourselves] to your own husbands as [a service] to the Lord. For the husband is head of the wife as Christ is the head of the church, Himself the Savior of [His] body.*

Cleave (*dabaq*) in Hebrew means "to adhere, to be glued, to stick; to be attached; soldering, welding together." It is a process and takes time; it certainly does not happen overnight. My husband and I still are being glued together, attached, and welded together. Have you ever seen anything being welded together? If steel, etc. could talk, I am sure while it is being welded together, it would yell "ouch!" Coming together as one definitely hurts! God is unifying us and making us one flesh. One flesh that is unselfish and humble and "each-other centered" and no longer self-centered.

Jesus' ultimate goal for married couples is to become one flesh. After more than thirty-six years of marriage, Reggie and I finish each other's sentences. We can pretty much tell you how the other will answer most questions. If we forget to tell each other that we are both going to the grocery store, both of us will come home with the same items. When he is hurting, I hurt and vice versa. Wives, do not get discouraged or frustrated because this "cleaving" does not happen even in a few years nor does it come easily or pain-free. Both of you must yield yourselves to the Holy Spirit to ensure that this "oneness" takes place.

Cleaving hurts! God is "smoldering" off the negative attributes in me and in my husband in order to make us more like Christ. Who wants to change? Who even thinks they need to change? Who wants to give up our selfish ways? None of us. I certainly did not. However, my husband and I have to change because we have a strong desire to reflect a Godly marriage to our daughters, granddaughter, church family and others. We want to exemplify how much God loves His Bride—the Church. Reggie and I long to make each other happy. We both realize that there is absolutely no need being married and unhappy. If you are going to be married, each spouse needs to learn how to make the other happy. And, you can learn to, if you want to learn. Reggie and I made a vow to love each other in sickness and in health, in good times and in bad, whether he is bald or has hair and whether or not gravity has taken over certain parts of my body!

In Genesis, God illustrates for us that in marriage male and female symbolically become one flesh. This is a supernatural blending of the hearts and lives of the married couple. All through the Bible, God treats this extraordinary relationship seriously. The aspirations in marriage should be more than companionship, love or lust; it should be oneness and a shared love for God. God gave marriage as a gift to Adam and Eve. Marriage was not just for convenience, friendship or lust. It was instituted by God.

When we see a happily married couple, we tend to think that there exists some mysterious blend of the "right" two people having been blessed to marry. Then, when we see an unhappy couple, we tend to think that those two people were simply "wrong" for each other. Sometimes that is all true. However, more often than not, marital relationships that are strained and battered occur when one or both partners do not understand that no human can make another whole and complete. With that being said, let us take a look at Myth #2: "Marriage Will Complete Me."

Lay Bare Your Soul . . . Expose yourself to the truth!
"Behold, You desire truth in the inner being; make me therefore to know wisdom in my inmost heart."
—Psalms 51:6

If you are single, are there any adjustments that you need to make to better prepare yourself for marriage? If you are married, can you identify any behaviors in which you partake that are detrimental to your relationship with your spouse? Examples: selfishness; stubbornness; withdrawal of affection.

_____
_____
_____
_____

What can you do today to improve your marriage?

_____
_____
_____
_____

Are you receiving the nourishment and life offered by Christ, the vine?

_____
_____
_____
_____

Are you abiding in Christ by:
- believing He is the Son of God? (I John 4:15)

- welcoming Jesus Christ as Lord of your life? (John 1:12)
- developing a mutual relationship with Christ? (I John 3:24)
- loving your husband as Jesus loves you? (John 15:12)

_____
_____
_____
_____

Myth #2: Marriage Will Complete Me

At a women's conference, I was speaking about building a healthy self-esteem and had mentioned this myth. After the session, a young woman came up to me timidly and asked if she could talk with me a few moments. I sensed that she needed more than just a few minutes so I asked if she could stay so we could talk alone. She eagerly agreed. When the hotel ballroom where I was speaking, finally emptied out, the young woman and I sat down; she then unexpectedly burst into tears.

She sobbed, "I am one of those women you spoke about earlier. Sometimes I feel like half a person. I am always saying how my fiancée completes me. Your words really hit home for me. I do not always love myself or my past behaviors in other relationships, but my husband-to-be will make me feel whole."

She continued to divulge to me about being raped by an older cousin at an early age and always thinking it was her fault. She had been promiscuous in previous relationships. However, since being born again and accepting the Lord as her personal Savior, she had been chaste. She knew God had forgiven her but she could not truly forgive her cousin or herself even though she tried to for years. Sometimes she felt like half a person—never quite fully complete.

Here I was sitting across from a beautifully dressed, lovely young woman whose image of herself had been negatively altered by an abuse, an attack on her body, her innocence, on her very soul. In the short time we spent together, I let her cry. Then I let her know that the rape was not her fault. I said that to truly love herself as God intended and feel whole she must forgive her attacker and herself for her past. I expressed to her that the abuse, in all likelihood, led her to be promiscuous because she no longer valued the sexual experience as being beautiful and reserved for marriage. I also put into words as lovingly as possible that it would be difficult to love her fiancée if she did not love herself. Loving yourself as God loves you is key to feeling complete and whole. We often enter marriage thinking that our husbands will complete whatever is lacking in ourselves.

I also related to her that she must find a way of dealing with her anger and resentment toward her attacker. If she continued to deny that anger and harbor resentment, she would always be in danger of sinning herself. In Hebrews 12:14–16 (AMP) it states:

> Strive to live in peace with everybody and pursue that consecration and holiness without which no one will [ever] see the Lord. Exercise foresight and be on the watch to look [after one another], to see that no one falls back from and fails to secure God's grace [His unmerited favor and spiritual blessing], in order that no root of resentment [rancor, bitterness, or hatred] shoots forth and causes trouble and bitter torment, and the many become contaminated and defiled by it—that no one may become guilty of sexual vice, or become a profane [godless and sacrilegious] person as Esau did, who sold his own birthright for a single meal.

Resentment arrives at the door of our hearts when we permit regret to deliver to us a bouquet of bitterness, animosity and hate or when we allow grudges over past hurts to appear at the doorstep of our minds. Resentment carries with it envy, rebellion, and sin. In spite of this, when we let the Holy Spirit saturate our hearts and minds, He can cure the damage that causes resentment.

I asked her, "Have you forgiven your cousin who wronged you?" If she could forgive her cousin, she would open herself to recovery, renewal, growth, and wholeness. I reminded her of Matthew 6:14–15 which states,

For if you forgive people their trespasses [their reckless and willful sins, giving up resentment], your heavenly Father will also forgive you. But if you do not forgive others their trespasses [their reckless and willful sins, leaving them, letting them go, and giving up resentment], neither will your Father forgive you your trespasses.

—(Amplified)

An innocent saying, "he's my better half," misleads us to believe that the two halves (husband and wife) will make a whole, complete person. Jane Hansen, president of Aglow International, says:

> When a woman's heart is turned—when she sets her desire back on God—a new freedom comes. The grasping in her voice and her attitude goes. She is able to move into relationship with members of the opposite sex based on wholeness rather than inappropriate neediness, hurt, and woundedness. As a wife, she is able to speak into her husband's life with more effectiveness because her worth and identity no longer depend on his response. When the woman stops looking to her husband for the needs he cannot meet, she frees him to meet the ones he can: the need for intimacy and shared responsibility for the marriage and family.

Explaining that there was no going back, I prayed with this young woman and I had her pray for herself. At long last she said she felt much better and she promised to walk in the forgiveness of God and know, by faith that she had forgiven her attacker. As a final point I encouraged her to seek a Christian women's support group for rape victims.

I am always mortified to learn of how many women of all races and backgrounds have been raped, molested or abused by men including their own fathers, brothers, cousins, uncles, ministers, and the list goes on and on. I ache for their sufferings and pray for God's manifested healing for them.

There are many other underlying factors that could cause you to feel like half a person, incomplete and unlovable. Besides abuse, maybe you experienced parental insults, neglect, rejection or parents who were overbearing and cold. Unresolved trauma suffered as a child or even as an adult can destroy a marriage in record time.

The main advice I can offer to single women is to deal with the devilish imps from your past before even contemplating marriage. Work on yourself. Seek competent, professional, Christian counseling. Become whole. The saying, "He's my better half" is a myth. No, let's be real. It is a lie! Each spouse must enter into marriage as whole individuals, not halves.

As first lady Serita Jakes says in her book, *The Princess Within*:

> A princess doesn't need to go to the mirror and ask, "who's the fairest of us all?" She understands that her worth is defended by all the soldiers in her Father's kingdom. She doesn't need to feel like she is the most beautiful or the most talented in all the land. She knows her value is not based on her own performance but is based on who her Father is. Her value is inherited and is unconditional. Although she can change what she does, nothing can change who she is—the precious daughter of the King.

What about loneliness? Quite a few women believe the myth that marriage will complete them because they will no longer be lonely. Well let me tell you, loneliness is an equal opportunity ailment. Whether single or married, young or not so young, white or black, we all have seasons of loneliness. Marriage is no cure-all for loneliness. Read this epistle of loneliness sent to me by a young married woman . . .

Dear Dr. Cynthia,

When I was 20 years old I was intensely pursued by a tall, well-mannered, dynamic guy with a bubbly sense of humor. He cared for me like a queen. When he proposed marriage I could not picture ever being alone or unhappy again. So, what took place after the wedding was quite alarming to me.

I discovered that I was only acquainted with a small fraction of my new husband's persona. I was extremely distressed when I discovered that my spouse was going to spend most of his free time watching TV. I was dreadfully disenchanted to find out that he did not like to cuddle, and I was not going to be held through the night, as I had dreamed. As a matter of fact, I am not even hugged tenderly, unless he is "in the mood." The wonderful wooing has died. As a newlywed, I can now only bawl in secret.

—Lonely Newlywed

Loneliness in marriage comes in all forms but the most common is when the husband is emotionally detached from his wife.

The husband may work hard, bring home his paycheck, have sex with his wife every so often but still be emotionally detached. He does not communicate on a deeper level, he does not re-affirm his wife, he does not touch or hold her (unless sexual intercourse is involved), he does not express his feelings, and on and on and on. If this describes your husband, you probably cannot remember the last time you went on a date and he treated you like he was madly in love with you and talked into the wee hours of the morning about everything.

Emotional detachment in a marriage is painful. You get married thinking: *I will have a close friend and lover for life. We will do everything together (at least, most things). I will just melt every time I see him and he will have a big grin on his face every time I walk in the room.* Well, it really can be like that but first you and your husband must banish the demons called "emotional detachment" lurking in your marriage.

I liken those "emotional-detachment demons" to the toy

called "jack-in-the-box." Have you ever played with a jack-in-the-box? You turn the handle and it plays music; when the music stops, the clown's head pops out of the top of the box. To start over, you press the clown's head down into the box and close the top.

Just imagine your husband never dealing with issues from his childhood or adulthood and constantly pressing those issues further and further down inside himself. Those issues could range from rejection, abandonment to abuse. When you seek intimacy from your husband, the clown's head—an issue—pops out, but without dealing with the issue, he simply stuffs it back inside himself.

Have you prayed and asked God to help you select a private time when you can discuss this with your husband? Tell your husband how much you love him and care how he feels. Tell him that you feel he must be trying to deal with a past issue that is hindering the intimacy in your marriage. Speak love, healing and acceptance to him. Assure him that he can share anything with you and you will not judge him nor tell anyone what he shares with you. (Then, keep your promise!) Encourage him to share that hurtful past with a trusted counselor or pastor. Offer to go with him. Tell him again how much you love him and want your marriage free of those issues popping up keeping you and him from bonding in a healthy way.

Do you want to be closer friends with your spouse? Let me give you some questions to ponder. Do you feel like you are not friends with your husband? Are you lonely for an emotional bond with your husband? What are you to do? First, you need to sit down with your husband and express how you feel and what you need from him. Be specific. Do not say you want more intimacy; say exactly what you want. More hand holding, more kissing, more hugging that is not foreplay for making love. Tell him you want an hour every day to talk about your dreams and his dreams, goals, failures, plans, and anything else you two want to talk about. Tell him you want a set date-night with just him once a month, or once a week. Whatever you both think is truly doable, do it and stick to it.

Loneliness in marriage can also come when you fall into the trap that your husband has to be your only friend. You should have a trusted girlfriend. You do not need many! One or two faithful, trusted girlfriends are more than enough. In the Amplified Bible, Proverbs 18:24 states:

> *The man of many friends [a friend of all the world] will prove himself a bad friend, but there is a friend who sticks closer than a brother.*

We all need friends who will stick close, care and be a present help when it is needed—in sunshine and in rain. It is healthier emotionally and spiritually to have one or two such friends than dozens of shallow acquaintances. Instead of trying to find one or two genuine friends, seek to develop into a friend. There are individuals who need your companionship. Ask God to show them to you, and then take on the challenge of being a genuine friend.

In addition to having one or two trusted girlfriends, learn to like being alone. Alone does not mean lonely. Alone, from an optimistic and constructive slant and style, means unique. Take yourself on a trip. And by trip I don't mean "trippin' " as in going out of your mind. And I don't necessarily mean taking a cruise that you cannot afford. Think outside the box. What about a day trip to a museum, the beach, or go to a movie? Join a woman's book club or woman's group at your church. Get a hobby. In essence, get a life!

"Lonely Newlywed" could not conceive of ever being lonely or unhappy again. What a tall tale! I frequently say to single women that they won't make good spouses for anyone in marriage if they can't be good to themselves first. Care for your psyche, body and spirit. Leaf through a paperback at your neighborhood bookstore, take a relaxing soak in the bathtub complete with bubbles, listen to your favorite tunes on your iPod, take a stroll around the neighborhood, PRAY, get in touch with your feelings in your journal, get pleasure from a much loved activity, go out to a film or a musical. And yes, you can go out by yourself!

As women, we get so little self-care time these days, and I promise you that any married woman, and specifically those with kids, would be tickled to have a late afternoon to focus only on their own needs!

Jesus, a single guy, regularly went off by himself to pray and break away from the demands of others and the stresses of the times. He is not a bad example to admire!

There is nothing immoral with having a desire for a spouse, but focusing solely on that seldom causes the guy to come out of hiding! Take the spotlight off of your wants and wishes and concentrate on others. It is in giving that we get. Volunteer your time, pay attention to the needs of relatives, classmates and friends and notice what happens. I promise you will soon encounter the intimacy of friendship and of service to others, rather than putting your whole existence on hold until that good-looking guy comes alongside you.

Talk to God about your thoughts and ask what this stage of what you designate as "loneliness" has to teach you. Chat with friends, members of the clergy, or spiritual advisers and ask for their assistance and encouragement.

Remember, a spouse does not have the capacity or capability to make the other spouse complete. A person's sense of completeness must come from God and no one else. In addition, do not fall into the trap of thinking you are going to change your husband. Let us examine the fallacies of Myth #3: "I Can Change Him!"

Lay Bare Your Soul . . . Expose yourself to the truth!

> *"Behold, You desire truth in the inner being; make me therefore to know wisdom in my inmost heart."*
>
> —Psalm 51:6

Did you suffer abuse as a child?

_____
_____
_____
_____

Were you neglected or abandoned?

_____
_____
_____
_____

Were you ever rejected?

_____
_____
_____
_____

Have you ever had an abortion?

_____
_____
_____
_____

Have you dealt with the wounds of your past?

How have you dealt with your past?

Have you forgiven the abusers?

Have you forgiven yourself?

How do you handle the moments of loneliness that arise in your life and/or marriage?

Can you discuss loneliness with your friends, family, spouse?

Myth #3: I Can Change Him!

Donald and Karla met in school while both were graduate students and every one of their acquaintances believed they were wonderful for each other. They were both young professionals and had bright futures. Donald grew up in a house where the dad was lord and master, often witnessing his dad hit his mom, and the family by no means questioned dad's ways. Donald consequently developed anger management issues from his family tree.

Karla graduated from school with a graduate degree and she had a great career. She came from a close family and as children they were encouraged to express their opinions. Karla, as a result, is extremely opinionated and speaks exactly what she feels which Donald finds rude.

Attracted to each other, Donald and Karla dated with the plan of getting married a year after their engagement. Almost immediately after the engagement, Donald's anger issues started to materialize, but rather than deal with the problems, all focus was on the wedding ceremony and the problems were relegated to a two hour pre-marital meeting with the pastor. As you can guess, the anger issue was swept under the rug as the pair prepared for the marriage ceremony.

Karla believes that now that they have been married for two months she can change him and the anger issue will be solved. You see, Karla's strategy during the time of engagement was that she would get what she wanted once they were married. The first month of marriage was grand but soon the ecstasy and joy started to diminish. In spite of this, Karla is determined to change her man!

I cannot begin to tell you how many times I have heard women say that about their husbands in the early years of marriage. I have also heard single women echo these very words before they walk to the altar. Ladies, what you see, is what you get! Single ladies, take the blinders off and truly see him. Is he always late? Does he make promises he does not keep? Is he always saying he will go on a diet tomorrow? Does he prefer his rather casual, sometimes unkempt appearance (and you want a sharp, debonair dresser)? Is he rude to his Mom (he may in turn be rude to you)? Does he not pay child support nor see his children regularly and consistently? Does he go from job to job? What if you are already married and now you want to change him like Karla?

Well, dear sister, only the Holy Spirit can significantly change another person, if and only if, he wants to change. To start with, it is crucial to realize and completely grasp that the responsibility of changing another human being is a duty that falls under the authority of the Holy Spirit, not another human being.

In the early years of marriage, I was particularly guilty of "trying to be the Holy Spirit" in my husband's life. It was a constant struggle against my flesh to keep myself from trying to tell him the "best" way to do things. **You see, I thought "my way" was always the "best way"! How egocentric!**

Even now, I can always tell when I am pushing too hard, when he says to me: "Honey, I need you to be my wife." In other words, I need to support him, back him, encourage him, let him know I am available to help him (if he wants my help). I do not need to organize him, manage him, mother him, nor nag him. He is an intelligent, grown man who truly loves the Lord and seeks the Lord every day (sometimes several times a day) so when he needs my help, he will ask.

To engaged couples, please pay attention. Recognize that

whatever flaws or dislikes you observe in your future spouse more often than not don't change in marriage within your own power. Even if the love of your life decides to change, it might take a while. If there are flaws that you cannot live with and you become aware of it prior to marriage, think seriously before getting into that marriage. NEVER go into marriage with the air of arrogance that you will change him.

Before we go further, let us examine Donald and Karla's relationship before marriage. We learned that almost immediately after their engagement, Donald's anger issues surfaced. Karla did not deal with this huge challenge in their relationship as soon as she recognized it.

Donald apparently learned to be "lord and master" from his dad. Donald also learned that it was acceptable to hit your wife because he saw his dad hit his mother. The only way Donald will deal with his anger issues is to acknowledge that he first, has a problem and second, wants to change.

I counsel many women who are nagging, begging and threatening their husbands to change. Do you think these husbands change simply because of their wives begging? No, indeed! However, when the husbands make a conscience decision that they need and want to change, they do. Of course, you can do something very critical, very important and very necessary—pray. I know you thought I was going to reveal an undiscovered secret. Well, my precious sister, that is the most important, critical and necessary thing you can do.

If Donald is physically abusive to Karla, she does not need to live with abuse. She needs to get out of that home and then pray for Donald. If Donald is verbally abusive, Karla needs to decide, and decide early, if she is going to accept that behavior from Donald. Many women have several children first, and then want to address their husband's anger issues. By then, the wives are suffering from low self-esteem, financially dependent on the husbands and afraid to leave. I do not advocate that any woman live with a husband who is abusing her. Seek wise counsel.

To influence change in your spouse with the help of the Holy Spirit,

TAKE IT TO GOD IN PRAYER. Pray that the Holy Spirit will bring about the needed change in your spouse.

DON'T NAG, PESTER OR ATTEMPT TO PUSH THE PERSON TO CHANGE.

UNDERSTAND THE ROOT OF THE BEHAVIOR.

Understanding the root of your husband's behavior, takes a great deal of prayer, observation of him and talking with him. When you seek God in prayer, ask the Holy Spirit to reveal to your husband the "root" causes of his behavior. The roots, like most plants, are deep under the surface and hidden. This will be a much different prayer than any you have probably even prayed. When you have a pure heart—no agenda to manipulate your husband—and pray that God help your husband, then the Holy Spirit can move.

Pray and believe:

> Lord, I repent for trying to change my husband. Only you know him because you made him. Lord, please help me to be more compassionate and understanding toward my husband. Change me; work on me to become the wife you want me to be. Please help my husband to understand why he acts the way he does. Reveal the root causes of his behavior to him. Reveal to him what only you can; cleanse him, wash him with the Blood of Jesus and help him to be the man and husband you want him to be. I believe you are the Great I Am. I give you all the praise, honor and glory, in Jesus' name. AMEN.

Then, observe your husband. "Be quick to listen and slow to speak." (James 1:19 NIV) When your spouse talks with you, does he believe that his viewpoints and thoughts are valued? Visualize a mental wristwatch and keep track of how much you speak and how much you listen. When we chatter too much and listen too little, we convey to our husbands that we assume our thoughts are of greater magnitude than theirs.

"Listen" carefully with your eyes and observe your husband interacting with people in different situations. Ask the Lord to open your husband's eyes to his own behavior. Once you have made numerous observations and have prayed about what you perceive, wait and ask God when the best time is to discuss your observations and perceptions. Remember, they are your perceptions, not necessarily his perceptions. Ask the Lord to remove judgment and your own stuff from your perceptions.

Have you observed your husband interacting with his family? Family interactions are the most telling and the most important. Do his parents (or people he grew up with) argue instead of communicate? Is his mother domineering and argues with your husband or doesn't let him get a word in? Does his mother treat him like a child? Does his father treat him as if he were invisible? Or, was his father in his life? There are hundreds of other observations you could make about how he interacts with his family. Ask yourself questions about his interactions with different people: with his children, with you, with his co-workers, etc. Does your husband blame others for his behavior(s)? Or, does he take the blame for everything even when he had nothing to do with the situation? Take all these questions to the Lord in prayer. Ask God to help you organize your thoughts into about two major questions at a time, then pray and wait on the Lord.

Whenever you feel the Lord urging you, talk with your husband about two major questions at a time. Do not spout off twenty questions at him at once. That is too overwhelming and may put him on the defensive. Be sure the timing is right, then say something like: "Honey (or whatever your pet name is for him), last week I observed how your Mom interacts with you. Has your Mom always been argumentative? How do you feel about that type of interaction?" If he doesn't answer, say, "Honey, I know you may need to think about what I have asked but would you promise me that we will talk about this later?" Trust God to help your husband to understand how his past is affecting his present behavior.

***Wait** on the **LORD**; be of good courage, And He shall strengthen your heart; **Wait**, I say, on the **LORD**!*
—Psalms 27:14

Waiting on God is not simple. Frequently it seems that He is not resolving our requests or does not grasp the importance of our circumstances. That sort of assessment means that God is not in charge or does not care. God is worth waiting for when it comes to your husband and your marriage. God uses waiting to revitalize and recharge us. Make use of your waiting periods by discerning what God may be trying to show you.

When you and your husband do discuss those questions, then ask him several more:

"How do you think the anger you experienced growing up is affecting you now?"

"How do you feel your behavior is affecting our children?"

Your husband, no matter what the root causes of his behavior, can change in the acceptance of your love. Rejection is often the basis for many behaviors.

I have had to learn to mirror acceptance to my husband. Did you know that you are a mirror to your spouse? What does he see when he looks into your eyes and when he reads your body language? If he sees lack of trust, disgust, lack of support, and lack of acceptance in your face and body language, it speaks volumes to him. If he sees rejection of him and what he does, the result will be fear. If he does not think you believe in him, he will fear rejection. The fear of rejection is one of the powerful forces controlling people today.

I John 4:18 (AMP) says:

There is no fear in love [dread does not exist], but full-grown (complete, perfect) love turns fear out of doors and expels every trace of terror! For fear brings with it the thought of punishment, and [so] he who is afraid has not reached the full maturity of love [is not yet grown into love's complete perfection].

Fear will begin to dissolve under a steady stream of supportive, encouraging, unconditional love.

I married my husband because his character showed me that he is responsible, dependable, mature, caring, generous, patient, and a man of his word. Therefore, after we discuss an issue and he says he will do something, I need to trust and believe that he will do it. I offer my help but if he does not need or want it, I believe that he can and will do what he said. He knows that I trust and believe that he will do what he says. I also know now that he will not do things the way I do and that is perfectly okay.

I liked his little idiosyncrasies before we got married and I have learned to still like them. Allow me to let you in on a note I received from a wife who was embarrassed by her husband's habits and unconventional behaviors . . .

Dear Dr. Cynthia,

My husband and I have been married for five years. Sometimes he embarrasses me so much when we are in public. He is so loud—he laughs and talks loud. Sometimes he even says inappropriate things to people which truly is embarrassing to me. For example, he might ask a lady if she's pregnant (and she's not—she's heavy). I know he does not mean to hurt anyone but he embarrasses me. What should I do?

Truly,
Mortified and Uncomfortable Wife

My reply . . .

Dear Mortified and Uncomfortable Wife,

Sweetie, my best advice for you is—you must be you and your husband must be himself. He certainly did not just start behaving like this; I am sure he behaved the same way before you were married. Did that behavior bother you then? Have you ever just had a delicate conversation with him about his behavior?

Have you ever thought that maybe this is more your problem than his problem? Why does his behavior bother you so much? Ask the Lord to reveal the answer to you.

I have learned if my husband's behavior is annoying to me, it means there is something in me that the Lord needs to work on in me. Consequently, I am learning to be more accepting, non-judgmental, and tolerant. I am also learning that Cynthia is Cynthia and my husband is himself. He cannot be me and I cannot be him.

Oftentimes, a genuine female friend can help you see your own behavior that may make you either judgmental of your spouse or too accepting of his abusive behaviors. Let us examine Myth #4: "No More Single Girlfriends for Me . . . I's Married Now!"

Lay Bare Your Soul . . . Expose yourself to the truth!
"Behold, You desire truth in the inner being; make me therefore to know
wisdom in my inmost heart."
—Psalms 51:6

Are you recognizing abusive behaviors in your spouse? If so, what types of conduct is being exhibited?

_____
_____
_____
_____

Is your husband willing to go to counseling? Why or why not?

Are you willing to go to counseling? Why or why not?

What does the Lord say to you about living with this abuse?

Maybe your husband is not abusive but has idiosyncrasies. What can you do to be less judgmental?

"Truly See Me" Prayer

Lord, help me to concentrate on my own behavior, thoughts and "STUFF." Lord, I seek you to help me. I believe that the same Holy Spirit that works in me can work in my husband. I cannot change my husband. Lord, bless us. Your will be done on earth in our lives as it is in heaven. In the name of Jesus Christ, I pray.
AMEN

Myth #4: No More Single Girlfriends for Me . . . I's Married Now!

Let us discuss genuine friendships with women first before we examine Myth #4.

Genuine, wholesome friendships with women—single or married—are always a blessing. In friendships, we should learn to be honest, trustworthy, loyal, offer constructive criticism and encouragement, be supportive, listen attentively, stand by her through the good and the bad. Sounds a lot like marriage, doesn't it? Friendships can certainly teach you a lot about yourself before you are married.

Proverbs 27:17 (NKJV) says:

Iron sharpens iron; so a man sharpens the countenance of his friends.

Female friendships can help you know who you are and what you are made of. Iron rubbed against iron shapes and sharpens it. So, constructive criticism between two friends can be a precious key to unlock who you really are; the hidden flaws in your character.

However, it also says in Proverbs 27:6:

Faithful are the wounds of a friend, but the kisses of an enemy are deceitful.

A friend who has your greatest wellbeing at heart may have to give you unpleasant advice at times, but you know it is for your own good. A friend's advice, no matter how painful, is much better. I can better appreciate the constructive criticism of a genuine girlfriend even though it may sting because she is being truthful in love than the kisses and lies of someone who is supposed to be my friend and stabs me in the back with vicious lies and gossip. Like many women, I have had girlfriends who were loyal and protected my secrets and helped me grow. I have also had girlfriends who stabbed me in the back because of their jealousy and their own insecurities.

Ladies, learn from your relationships with women. Those lessons will help you in marriage. You will learn how to value someone else's feelings, be supportive and encouraging, hold secrets to your heart, and learn compromise and other valuable lessons. In my twenties, I would say, "I would rather be friends with men than women, because women are so catty and petty." Well, not all women. We, as women, need the iron that sharpens iron in female relationships to help us see ourselves. So learn your lessons well. Trust me, when you are married, there will be a whole lot of iron sharpening going on!

On to the subject of married women having single girlfriends. Single or married, women would be well advised to pray and ask God for a friend. However, be sure to keep friends in their proper perspective. Do not put your friends before your husband. My friends do not come before my husband. Furthermore, I do not tell my girlfriends anything that I cannot tell my husband. My husband is my best friend.

I counsel many women who share everything with their girlfriends and nothing with their husbands. Then, they wonder why they are not close to their husbands. There are many things I have shared only with my husband.

I am not an insecure person; however I do have common sense. Common sense dictates that, as a married woman, you do not leave your girlfriend (single or married) alone with your husband.

Ask God to send you a few girlfriends who will enjoy some good old fashioned company. A buddy who you can go walking with, meet for chocolate or dinner once in a while, work out with at the gym, go SHOPPING! Married women need female friends for their coffee breaks, morning walks, sharing errands and chores or even to celebrate a birthday. Have a "Girl's Night Out" every so often. It will keep you sane! I know from experience; it is so much fun and you will look forward to it. Nothing is better than having some time with those friends that can make you grin and giggle!

Female friends let married women take time off from being "Supermom" and "SuperSpouse." They can be women and share concerns with each other that they cannot hardly ever chat with others about because of everyday happenings in life. Our friendships, which I will also call "shared connections," are very important to our emotional well–being. From time to time, married women get so bogged down in caring for our household, husband, career and other tasks that our girlfriends may be the lone folks who can reach us and let us decelerate.

Girlfriends share our experiences, tell us jokes and pay attention to our stories. You need girlfriends. The need for these "shared connections" does not diminish our married relationships by any measure. We need all of these different interactions for diverse reasons.

I also want to caution women on the number of girlfriends you have as a married woman. In the early years of marriage, I only had time for one girlfriend who was also married. We really did not see each other a lot. We were busy with children, school, husbands, work and church.

When the children are older and the marriage has grown, there will be plenty of time for get-away weekend trips with your girlfriend. When the children are young, having another married couple with children as friends is fun and helps maintain the sanity.

Isn't it funny that we pray for everything but friends? Always remember to pray for a girlfriend and let God put you two together.

Here is a note I received from a wife who communicates more with her single girlfriend than her husband . . .

Dear Dr. Cynthia,

I have heard you speak a lot about "your husband is your best friend." I would love that too. My husband and I have been married for four years. I try talking with my husband and try sharing my hopes, dreams, and secrets. He is not very supportive or encouraging.

Therefore, I find myself still talking and sharing my dreams and secrets with my single girlfriend who is very encouraging. Am I wrong to continue to share with my single girlfriend when my husband is so unresponsive?

From the Bottom of My Heart,
Talk 2 Me

My answer?

Dear Talk 2 Me,

I sympathize with you. However, allow me to ask you these questions:

Does your husband, at least, listen to you?

Have you encouraged your husband to share his goals and dreams with you?

Are your expectations that your husband will respond just like your friend responds?

We must set the mood, if you will, when we want to have serious talks with our husbands. You cannot have deep discussions when he is distracted or tired. Try preparing him by saying something like this: "Honey (substitute your endearing name for your hubby), there has been something very pressing on my heart to share with you. I need your input on something I have been mulling over about my goals (or, whatever the topic is). When's a good time to talk with you?"

Then during the actual discussion, are you open to his opinions and advice? If he is not as communicative as you would like, try asking him these questions:

Have you ever had a goal like this one?

What are your wildest dreams?

One last word of advice: Do not expect your husband to respond like your girlfriend. Appreciate your husband's and your girlfriend's distinctly different responses. Learn to savor them both.

Finally, married women should understand another purpose for having single girlfriends. It is not just about getting a "social connection," emotional well being or a "Girl's Night Out." It is about giving single women advice, support and wisdom. In I Timothy 5, it states:

> *[Treat] older women like mothers [and] younger women like sisters, in all purity.*
>
> —(AMP)

When married women appreciate single women as fellow members in the family of God, they will watch over them and help them develop spiritual integrity. Having been married for more than thirty-six years, it is easy for me to disregard "the single life." As a married woman, there are things I can share with my single girlfriends.

When I was single, I HATED when my married girlfriends would advise me, "Oh, you will just KNOW when Mr. Right comes along." WHAT does THAT mean??!!?? That one declaration used to DRIVE ME WILD! Now that I am married, I recognize things that I never understood as a single woman. I really think that there is a big chasm stuck between "the single life" and "the married life." I see that "the single life" is on one edge of "the great gulf" and "the married life" is countless miles away on the other edge. Single women shout from their edge fears, desires, doubts and needs in order to gain some Godly insight from their married girlfriends. However, once the girlfriend goes across "the great divide" by saying, "I do," the void stuck between the two sides is too pronounced. The opinions and replies are spoken, but in an unheard-of language that single women sometimes cannot translate. For example, as a married girlfriend may say to her single girlfriend, "Don't rush it! Benefit from your singleness! Now that I am married, there are oodles of stuff I wish I had done prior to getting married." Then, the well-intentioned married girlfriend will cite II Corinthians 7:25–28, 32–35 (The Message):

> The Master did not give explicit direction regarding virgins, but as one much experienced in the mercy of the Master and loyal to him all the way, you can trust my counsel. Because of the current pressures on us from all sides, I think it would probably be best to stay just as you are. Are you married? Stay married. Are you unmarried? Don't get married. But there's certainly no sin in getting married, whether you're a virgin or not. All I am saying is that when you marry, you take on additional stress in an already stressful time, and I want to spare you if possible.
>
> I want you to live as free of complications as possible. When you're unmarried, you're free to concentrate on simply pleasing the Master. Marriage involves you in all the nuts and bolts of domestic life and in wanting to please your spouse, leading to so many more demands on your attention. The time and energy that married people spend on caring for and nurturing each other, the unmarried can spend in becoming whole and holy instruments of God. I'm trying to be helpful and make it as easy as possible for you, not make things harder. All I want is for you to be able to develop a way of life in which you can spend plenty of time together with the Master without a lot of distractions.

Well, let me address married women: Don't quote this scripture to a single woman! First, let's make clear what Paul is suggesting. Paul saw the approaching maltreatment that the Roman regime would soon bring upon Christians. He gave this guidance because being single would mean less distress and more freedom to throw one's life into the cause of Christ (I Corinthians 7:29), even to the point of boldly dying for Him. Paul's counsel shows his single-minded zeal to spreading the Good News.

Okay, as Christians, whether married or single, we ought to be throwing our lives into the cause of Christ and be dedicated to spreading the Good News. However, let's be real. Even when a single woman is fully dedicated to spreading the Good News, more often than not, there is still a hint of an emotional skirmish going on because there is a longing to be married.

As a married friend, it is our responsibility to help our single friends discover what they believe about marriage and why they feel they are prepared to be married. Lots of single women innocently reason that marriage will answer all their troubles (economic security, on-demand sex, etc.) Well, my single friends, here are some problems marriage will not resolve:

- Loneliness
- Sexual temptation
- Removal of life's obstacles
- Fulfillment of one's deepest emotional needs.

Can I get an AMEN from the married women?!? As married women, I think God places single women in our lives so we can share our experiences, strength and faith with them. So, we should be sharing that marriage single-handedly does not keep two individuals together . . . commitment does. Commitment in marriage means being dedicated to Christ FIRST and then to each other (spouse-to-spouse) even with struggle and troubles. As amazing as marriage is, it does not automatically resolve all dilemmas. Whether married or single, we have to be satisfied with our situation and concentrate on Christ, not our spouse, to resolve our troubles.

We, as married women, should advise our Christian sisters who are single to not look upon marriage as an essential aim in life. Some of our single sisters experience incredible pressure to be married. From time to time, that unnecessary load comes from us well intentioned married women. We turn into matchmakers and think our single girlfriends are unappreciative when they are not interested in somebody we fix them up with from work. Married women, remember when you were single and HATED when a married friend (or family member) would try to fix you up with the guy from the company who was monetarily set but at forty was still living with a roommate?

Instead, as a married woman, share with your single girlfriends that life is not whole only with a spouse. Share that the reality is that when one gets married it does not suggest life is picture perfect; it is not.

As you can tell by what has been shared with you in this section, having a single girlfriend is not a terrible thing if you keep the relationship in proper perspective and comprehend the part you can play in helping a single sister appreciate life, relationships and the significance of placing marriage in its proper perspective. Girlfriends are very important for all women. Female friendships are critical commodities for married women. With girlfriends, whether married or single, these are the friends we can take the time to let down our hair, let down our guard, crack jokes, be ourselves, and relax.

As much as you understand the importance of one or two trusted, genuine girlfriends who you will have to build up and encourage sometimes, let us look at the importance of building up your husband in Myth #5: "It's Not My Job to Build Him Up!"

Lay Bare Your Soul . . . Expose yourself to the truth!
"Behold, You desire truth in the inner being; make me therefore to know
wisdom in my inmost heart."
—Psalms 51:6

Do you have one or two trusted, genuine girlfriends? If no, why not? If yes, identify them and list why they are genuine girlfriends.

_____
_____
_____
_____

Have you been hurt by females in the past? If your response is yes, have you forgiven them? If you have not forgiven them, clarify why.

_____
_____
_____
_____

What does the Bible say about forgiveness?

_____
_____
_____
_____

What characteristics are you looking for in a genuine girlfriend?

_____
_____

Do you exemplify those same characteristics? If not, what will you do to grow?

Myth #5: It's Not My Job to Build Him Up!

Have you asked yourself these questions?

> Have you ever been puzzled by your husband's lack of confidence?
> Why is my husband driven toward super achievement?
> Or, why is my husband so apathetic about life?
> Why is he so passive; so indecisive?
> Why does my husband have difficulty admitting fault or asking for forgiveness?
> Why is my husband so preoccupied with his past?
> And, why is he guarded in relationships? Even our own?

All these questions represent an erosion in self-confidence; an erosion of a healthy self-image. Your husband may appear to have it altogether, but you know, as few others do, that underneath that self-sufficient exterior lives a man who needs to be built up. We all need to be built up and accepted and loved unconditionally but as the scripture says in Proverbs 14:1 (NKJV):

> *A wise woman builds her house, but the foolish pulls it down with her hands.*

Wives, our responsibilities are to **build up** our husbands, not tear them down. For your husband to begin to respond to you in a more open, loving way, you are going to have to accept him just as he is; not for what you hope he will become. Your unconditional love may be the first he has received from a significant adult. He may not have received it from parents, grandparents, teachers, and especially from male role models.

Some of the most seemingly potent artillery in Satan's armory are mental weapons. Perhaps his best mental weapon is low self-worth. Low self-worth is having a low view of oneself whether it is a feeling of incompetence where we don't fit a certain standard we have set for ourselves or an opinion of feeling unwanted.

My husband and I counsel so many couples where the fear of rejection is running rampant in their marriages. If you want your husband's self-esteem strengthened, then begin to recognize and pray against that fear of rejection. In I John 4:18 we know that "perfect love casts out fear." Fear will begin to dissipate under the steady stream of genuine love. Getting your love will calm his fears and give him self-confidence.

How do you "build up" your husband? If you are sincere and persistent and consistent in faithfully using the following five easy and powerful tools, you will begin to notice a positive difference in your man's self-confidence and self-worth:

PRAY FOR HIM. You will need to pray to God for wisdom. God says in the Book of Proverbs if you want wisdom, simply ask Him for it. It takes wisdom to have a successful marriage. You will need insight into your husband's personality that only God can give you. Consecrate your husband by praying for him. The Apostle Paul instructed all Christians to pray for one another in Ephesians 6:18. Make immediate, short prayers your regular reaction to each situation that involves your husband during the day. You don't have to isolate yourself from other people and from everyday work in order to pray continually for your husband. Sincere and heartfelt prayer for your husband is good for him, for you and the "holy healthiness" of your house. Do you recognize that Satan desires to devastate and damage your spouse, particularly his spirit, moral fiber and his headship in your relationship? Have complete confidence in God through prayer as you daily surrender your husband and marriage to the wise, loving care of the Lord Jesus.

PRAISE HIM. Every man needs his wife to accept him for who he is and not for what she wants him to be. He also wants his spouse to value and appreciate him. Accept him and appreciate him. How many people at work tell your husband: "Great job." "You're so smart." "You're right."—probably very few, if any. As his wife, you *must* tell him: "good idea," "good choice," "you're absolutely correct, honey," as often as you possibly can. Men must have their egos built up. And, if we are not careful, wives, we will tear them down. Praise your husband with public displays of admiration. Shower him with thank you notes, hugs, smiles, and calls to show gratitude for all that he is in your life.

PAMPER HIM. Some husbands need more pampering than others. However, all husbands need to feel that they are the sparkle in the eyes of their own wife. Not only tell him how much you adore and love him but show him in as many little ways as you can. Rub the back of his neck while he's driving or watching television. Rub his feet, if he likes that. Write him little love and admiration notes and put them where he will find them. Make him feel like the king of his castle. The priest of his home. Make his home a place of refuge and peace and joy. A place where he rushes to in order to feel adored and welcomed and at peace. Don't rush him the moment he comes in the door with complaints and problems. Rush to the door and shout, "My honey's home!" and give him a big kiss. I do that every chance I get! When I read that Sarah called Abraham her "lord" out of respect and admiration, I started doing the same thing. No, he is not my "Lord" but he is my "lord": my husband, the father of our two daughters, the granddad of one granddaughter, he is my covering, he is the one I look to for support and care and encouragement, he provides for me and the girls, he is my lover; yes, Reginald Allen McGill is my "lord."

PROTECT HIS IDEAS, SECRETS AND GOALS. There is nothing more devastating to a man's ego than for him to finally share a piece of himself—his dreams, his past, his secrets and then we stomp on those fragile pieces of himself that he gave to us to protect. We should protect and pray about everything our husbands share with us. We are not to run and tell Momma, our girlfriends, or our children. Tell NO ONE BUT GOD! Remember, ladies, we are a mirror to our husbands and we should reflect acceptance and safety and protection. We are the "receiver" (as in sexual intimacy as well as in relational intimacy), so receive in love—without judgment, without condemnation. When you do that, he will keep sharing more and more and more with you. The two of you will become *best* friends!

PUBLICLY HONOR HIM. Of course, this is assuming that you privately honor him already. You must never criticize him in public nor in front of the children. A quick way to "tear down" your husband is to criticize, humiliate and undermine him in public. A publicly humiliated husband is hard to "build up" privately. Even in private, it is important to measure your words. Once something has been spoken, it is hard to pull it back. When you argue, never attack his character, always attack the problem. Study your own husband and see what works best for your relationship.

Building your mate's self-esteem is an integral part of your marriage. As you are building each other's self-esteem, you are truly learning to become husband and wife in the biblical sense. Genesis 2:24 states:

Therefore a man shall leave his father and his mother and shall be-

*come united and cleave to his wife **and they shall become one flesh.***
—Amplified Version

Matthew 19:4–5 states:

*He (Jesus) replied, Have you never read that He who made them from the beginning made them male and female, and said, For this reason a man shall leave his father and mother and shall be united firmly (joined inseparably) to his wife, **and the two shall become one flesh**?*
—Amplified Version

From these passages of scripture we come to understand that the male and female are united as one by taking responsibility for each other's well being and by loving the mate above all others.

Proverbs 14:1 says:

*Every **wise** woman **builds** her house, but the **foolish** one tears it down with her own hands.*

Webster's Dictionary defines "wise" as:

having the ability to discern or judge what is true, right or lasting; sagacious; exhibiting common sense; prudent; shrewd; crafty.

And, "foolish" is defined as:

lacking or exhibiting a lack of good sense or judgment; silly; unwise.

If your marriage is to thrive and grow, you will need to learn to become a wise woman. There were many times in the early years of my marriage when I was truly foolish. I said foolish words; I acted foolish; I thought fool heartedly. I can clearly see now how I was tearing my house down with my own words, thoughts and deeds.

Build, as implied in Proverbs 14:1 means to lay one brick upon another brick. Each brick in our marriage and in our home represents our relationships with our husbands, children, and others. What bricks are you laying in your marriage?

- Bricks of discord, jealousy, mean-spiritedness, cruelty, or
- Bricks of understanding, forgiveness, love, laughter and peace?

Women can be the greatest, most influential builders of happy marriages or we can foolishly tear our marital relationship apart brick by brick. Ladies, repeat after me, "It is my job to build up my husband. So therefore, I will, with God's direction and help."

You *can* boost the self-worth of your husband. To start with, you should identify where he needs bolstering. Lots of women are so caught up in finding their own identity that they make assumptions about the confidence of their husbands. Your husband may be grown-up on the exterior, but inside he absolutely has some lack of self-confidence. He may not be certain how to be a male in this race where women have increasing individualism and the populace is altering the conventional rules of relationships.

Seek to recognize why your spouse is acting a certain way. Focus on him, not on the negative circumstances and how you are affected. Perhaps he is subconsciously communicating by his actions some profound need for encouragement or allegiance.

I have observed or read about many married women throughout my thirty-six years of marriage and would like to share some of the lessons they have taught me. Here are just a few:

1. Eve
2. Job's wife

3. Queen Esther
4. My mother, Doris Herbin Tarpley

Eve

I have often asked myself, when you have it as good as Eve had it in the Garden of Eden (Genesis 2 & 3), why would she jeopardize all she had by being so foolish? The Garden of Eden was not only beautiful but a refuge, a place of shelter and safety where Eve and her husband, Adam, communed with God quite easily and with each other. There was no crime, no sadness, no washing dishes, no rivalry between husband and wife, just love and peace and joy, communing with God and communing with her husband. So why would a woman destroy such a union and relationship in such beautiful surroundings? The Bible clearly states that Eve was deceived by Satan in Genesis 3:13 with further explanations in II Corinthians 11:3 and I Timothy 2:14. Adam ate the forbidden fruit after God explicitly told him not to eat it.

The influence a wife has over her husband is phenomenal. Even *after* God forbade Adam to eat of the fruit of just one tree and even after Adam was closer to God than he ever could be his wife influenced him to do something he knew he should not have done. When God asked Adam why he ate of the forbidden fruit, he did not answer: "because I wanted to taste it"; nor did he reply, "because I just wanted to be 'the man' and do what I wanted to do." No, he answered God in Genesis 3:12 and said:

And the man said, The woman whom You gave to be with me—she gave me [fruit] from the tree, and I ate.
—Amplified Version

Women, we have too much influence over our husbands to use our influence unwisely!

Job's Wife

Let us now examine Job's wife (note that we never learn her name in the Bible) as I so often do to learn what *not* to do as a wife. Job's wife must have been under a great deal of stress not to have supported her husband during the time when catastrophic events befell both her and her husband.

Job's wife had a life of wealth and privilege and the Bible says Job was a righteous and well-respected man who truly feared and loved the Lord. However, when hardship falls, some women cannot stand the adversity that it brings. While hardship revealed Job's pure motives, they surfaced his wife's impure ones.

Satan's prediction to God was that if hardship befell Job, he would "surely curse You to Your face" (Job 1:11, 2:5). Is it coincidence that Job's wife echoes those same words? Job's own wife says: "Do you still hold fast to your integrity? Curse God and die" (Job 2:9). Often, it is the spouse who Satan will use to discourage and divert one's faith from God.

Job asked his wife:

*But he said to her, You speak as one of the impious and **foolish women** would speak. What? Shall we accept [only] good at the hand of God and shall we not accept [also] misfortune and what is of a bad nature?*

—(Amplified Version)

Job called his wife in that verse, a "foolish woman." Job's wife failed her husband when he needed her the most. How often have you failed your husband when he was at his lowest? Have you emasculated your husband with your harsh, insensitive words? Even when he made no sense at all but was hurting, did you comfort and encourage him or essentially just turn your back on him as Job's wife? Yes, you can be devastated and need comforting too but <u>sometimes</u> we must turn away from our feelings and be the stronger one and offer him words of encouragement.

I know I have been guilty of acting like Job's wife. I want my comfort and I want things my way but if my husband is facing some hardship, I need to put my own comfort aside and be there for him. Years ago, my husband was diagnosed with prostate cancer. A righteous man, an awesome, loving, caring husband, father and best pastor in the whole world—diagnosed with prostate cancer. He is such a man of faith. We told our family, close friends and the congregation that after much prayer, he believed God was going to heal him through surgery. He kept up a smile; kept right on preaching, teaching and counseling; kept right on seeing others healed as he laid hands on them and God healed them. However, I knew that he needed encouragement and comforting.

Even though he was consoling me, at times, I needed to be strong and activate my faith and encourage him. Needless to say, he is indeed fully healed and fully restored! Praise God!

Queen Esther

Queen Esther was truly a role model to us all of a truly wise woman. Esther, a displaced, orphan Jewess, had been reared by Mordecai, an older relative. She had been chosen in a beauty contest to be the Persian king's, King Ahasuerus's, new Queen out of many other lovely young ladies. Mordecai encouraged Esther to keep her religious heritage a secret for Persians did not intermingle with Jews.

Mordecai learned after King Ahasuerus married Esther that the Jewish people were to be killed by one of the King's trusted yet wicked officials, Haman. Haman was a self-promoting, evil man who elevated himself to vice-regent, second only to King Ahasuerus. Faced with a desperate challenge for survival for not only her own people but for herself as well, Esther pondered Mordecai's question:

> *For if you keep silent at this time, relief and deliverance shall arise for the Jews from elsewhere, but you and your father's house will perish. And who knows but that you have come to the kingdom for such a time as this and for this very occasion?*
> —Esther 4:14, Amplified Version

Courageously, Esther accepted the call. Interesting that Esther immediately decided to fast and pray before doing anything else. How many of us fast and pray when we want God to direct us, to save our loved ones, to move on our behalf? Esther did not barge in on the King and say, "Save my people!" As a matter of fact, no one was to enter the King's court unless he had summoned you; not even his wife—the queen.

Esther was a very wise woman and she sought God's direction in fasting and prayer. Then, she asked the King to see her. Yet, she still did not plead for her people. She invited her husband and evil Haman to dinner—not once—but twice before stating her plea.

After both meals and after her husband was relaxed and caught up in Esther's beauty and perfume and spoiling him, the King wanted to give Esther whatever she requested. Not until after the second dinner did Esther plead her cause and reveal her own heritage.

Divine guidance directed Esther's thoughts, words and actions. She won the respect and the ear of her husband. How many of us desire the respect and ear of our husbands? What have we done to earn that respect? The King assigned Queen Esther the task of rewriting the law (Esther 9:29) and thereby saving her people and herself.

Doris Herbin Tarpley

My Christian mother was and still is my most influential and important role model. What I have learned from her about being a loving, caring, wise wife is worth more than gold to me. My Mom and Dad were married for forty-eight years before he died. During his long illness with colon cancer, my mother cared for my father with the love, attention and care of a saint.

As a young girl, I did not understand why my Mom would do or say some of the things she did. I would whisper to myself or write in my diary, "I'll never let a man tell me what to do!" I did not understand why she "held her tongue" sometimes and would not argue with Dad. I did not understand why she would tell us four girls, "go ask your Dad about that." I did not understand why she would say to us, "just wait, be patient and let me talk to him about thus and so at the right time." I did not understand when she would say, "girls, learn to pick your battles; don't turn everything into a conflict."

After years of marriage, my Mom's words of wisdom, and role modeling would come back to me like pictures on television and then in the context of my marriage I would understand that sometimes it is better to "hold my tongue" and not argue with my husband. I may need to let him just say what is on his heart, while I remain silent. Take what he said in prayer. If God tells me to discuss that issue again then I will, but if God says, "leave it alone," then I must *leave it alone.* Oh, that is so hard sometimes!

Once we had two daughters of our own, I understood that sometimes our girls needed to go ask their Dad's permission to do thus and so. It was important that our daughters did not see me as the authority figure all the time. It was also important that they learned to respect their father so later they could learn to respect their Heavenly Father and then their own husbands.

As situations arose when my daughters would want me to "please ask Dad right now for me!", I learned to tell them, as my

Mom had told me, "let me talk with Dad at the right time. Now is not the right time." And, I did learn, as every married woman needs to learn, not to turn everything in your marriage into a battle.

My mother, like the Proverbs 31 wife, was praised by her husband.

> *A capable, intelligent, and virtuous woman—who is he who can find her? She is far more precious than jewels and her value is far above rubies or pearls. The heart of her husband trusts in her confidently and relies on and believes in her securely, so that he has no lack of [honest] gain or need of [dishonest] spoil. She comforts, encourages, and does him only good as long as there is life within her.*
>
> —Proverbs 31:10–12 (AMP)

> *Her children rise up and call her blessed (happy, fortunate, and to be envied); and her husband boasts of and praises her [saying], Many daughters have done virtuously, nobly, and well [with the strength of character that is steadfast in goodness], but you excel them all. Charm and grace are deceptive, and beauty is vain [because it is not lasting],* ***but a woman who reverently and worshipfully fears the Lord, she shall be praised!*** *Give her of the fruit of her hands, and let her own works praise her in the gates [of the city]!*
>
> —Proverbs 31:28–31 (AMP)

Why was the Proverbs 31 wife, Queen Esther, and my mother trusted and praised by their husbands? The answer can be found in verse 30b of Proverbs 31:

> ***but a woman who reverently and worshipfully fears the Lord, she shall be praised!***

When we reverence and fear the Lord, when we seek His eternal guidance and wisdom, when we fast and pray to Jesus

Christ and obey, then we can truly be wives that are respected and praised by our husbands.

In my early years of marriage, I often sulked and whispered to myself: "If Reggie were more like me, we wouldn't have this problem!" Let's look at Myth #6: "He Should Be More like Me!"

Lay Bare Your Soul . . . Expose yourself to the truth!
"Behold, You desire truth in the inner being; make me therefore to know wisdom in my inmost heart."
—Psalms 51:6

Pray that your husband will mature spiritually and ponder his responsibility before the Lord Jesus.

> God, help my husband to get to know you better and better. Help my husband to mature in the grace and knowledge of our Lord and Savior Jesus Christ. Help my husband to keep his heart with all vigilance, making sure that he concentrates on those desires that will keep him on the correct pathway. Help him to look directly to you, to keep his eyes set on the goals you have placed in his heart and not to get preoccupied on detours that lead to sin. Father, I thank you for the performance of it, in Jesus' name.
> —Prayer based on II Peter 3:18 and Proverbs 4:23–27

Pray that your husband's connection with God and His Word will bear fruit in his life.

> God, your Words says, "the fear of the Lord is the beginning of wisdom, and the knowledge of the Holy One is insight." I thank you that my husband acknowledges God as the foundation of wisdom. May my husband receive the blessings of honor, success, protection and freedom from worry as he trusts in You and delights in obeying Your commands. I thank you that my husband fears You, believes Your promises and willingly obeys You. I give you praise for it all, Father, in the name of Jesus Christ.
> —Prayer based on Proverbs 3:7, Proverbs 9:10 and Psalm 112:1

Pray that your husband will mature in headship in your marital relationship, caring and providing for you and your home.

> Lord, instruct my husband, according to your Word, to be willing to sacrifice for our family and to make our well-being of primary importance. Help me to surrender to his authority as he surrenders to Your authority. Help my husband to love me as You love the church. As his wife, help me to follow him as He follows You. Help me to cheer and support him. Grant my husband the emotional, intellectual and physical capacity to work hard and be just and fair-minded in all the affairs of life. Amen, and so be it.
> —Prayer based on Ephesians 5:25–29 and Colossians 3:19

Sit down with a pen and paper and make a list of all the strengths that your husband has as well as all the affirmative things that you can say about him. This could include skills he may have or attributes that he possesses. Include in this list all the positive things that you have ever heard people say about him.

Then, memorize and pronounce these strong points over your husband during your prayer time, over him while he naps and, when you feel comfortable, tell them to him openly. I promise that you will see your man transform before your very eyes! Here is an example:

My Husband

My husband is a gentleman and a gentle man.
My husband is confident.
My husband is my provider and my defender.
There is nothing my husband would not do for me.
My husband anticipates my needs and wants.
Every day my husband tells me and shows me how much he loves me.

I don't have to perform in order to deserve his love.
My husband honors all of his promises.
No one can change his opinion of me.
My husband is the ultimate intimate partner.
My husband cannot disown or divorce me because I am a part of him.
My husband covers me and doesn't expose me.

NOW THAT'S LOVE!

Now, your turn! Write your own special declaration prayer concerning your husband to pray over him.

_____
_____
_____
_____

Myth #6: He Should Be More Like Me!

Dear Dr. Cynthia:

My husband and I have only been married three months and the differences I now observe in my spouse are raising my blood pressure! Our individual routine and the traditions I grew up with are poles apart. I realize this may sound stupid, but, he squeezes the toothpaste tube in the middle, doesn't clean the bathtub after his shower, and does not fold up his underwear, after I labor to launder them, before placing them in the dresser drawer.

Why can't he be more like me?

—D2D (Distressed Due to Differences)

Dearest D2D:

No matter how similar you thought you and your husband were before marriage, you now have to understand that you won't always see eye to eye on every topic or matter. What you express in your letter is only the beginning! As your marriage continues, you will find you have even more conflicting views on things which directly disturb your marriage, such as child-rearing and money management.

Having differences of opinion doesn't make either of you wrong, just different. Differences are to be expected, but it doesn't have to be harmful to your marriage. Spouses have different points of view and ways of behaving centered in their upbringing and prior experiences. Those differences do not mean that one spouse is correct and the other incorrect, it just means they are not alike in their views or feelings.

Differences, when dealt with properly, can be good for your marriage in that fresh ideas and innovative ways of looking at things are presented to you and your husband and to your marriage. I recommend that you buy his and hers toothpastes. You have your own tube and he has his own. Tell him, "Honey, squeeze to your heart's content." Some things are just not worth getting your panties in a bunch. Spend a few more dollars and always have his and hers toothpastes available. Now, take a deep breath on this one. If he does not want to fold his clothes before he puts them in his dresser drawer, remember, those are his clothes—not your clothes. Now, the cleaning of the bathtub is probably very important to you so I suggest you place a cleaner and sponge right inside the tub on the ledge and tell your husband how important a clean tub is to you. Tell him that you clean the tub when you get out just for him and would really appreciate the same.

I have heard D2D and many other married women say, "I wish my husband was more like me." Do you really want that to become a reality? Or, do you want him to be more like Jesus?

Over thirty-six years ago, I wanted my husband to be more like me. Look up the word "perfectionist" in the dictionary and you will see my picture. Being a perfectionist has caused me to do a lot of self-reflection and self-discovery. I was the first-born and I simply loved to achieve. I was (and still am to an extent) an overachiever.

I wanted to do everything perfectly and furthermore, I wanted everyone else around me to be perfect too. I held myself to high standards as well as my husband. Just because I would finish a task days ahead of schedule, I would want him to do the same. Just because I want an orderly study, I would expect the same of him. He is not a slob, by any means, and he does complete tasks—just in his own timing and not in mine.

When we were first married, I wanted everything to be just so. The house spotless, the bed made in the morning, no dinner dishes left in the sink. I would even line up boots and shoes by the door. Nothing is wrong with wanting a clean house but an obsession is a totally different matter. I was obsessed. I wanted him to be as obsessive as I. When he rebelled, I did not understand. My obsessive, perfectionist behavior affected other areas of our marriage. I wanted him to be a "perfect" husband and do as I say do! NOT! What is a "perfect" husband anyway?

Have you met my husband? He is not to be bullied but he is about as perfect as they come. He is forgiving, caring, loving, responsible, communicative, attentive to me and much, much more! However, he became all that and even more when I released him to God. And, he wanted to be the husband God wanted him to be. Also, I had to fall on my knees and ask God to show me myself and ways I needed to change my past behavior.

The Bible says in Psalms 118:5 (NKJV):

I called on the Lord in distress; the Lord answered me and set me in a broad place.

God wants us to deal with the past and then put it behind us. Philippians 3:13–14 instructs us to forget what is behind (deal with it, forgive and then forget it). We must strain and press forward (sometimes it takes all the strength we can muster—with God's help) to move forward and not stay stuck in the past.

*My husband and I have only been married three months and the **differences** I now observe in my spouse are raising my blood pressure!*

Let's look at "**differences**" in marital relationships. There is good news and bad news. First, the bad news: When a man and a woman are in love with each other, differences and disputes will happen.

Now, the good news: A married couple does not have to end it all by launching a disastrous relationship battle or engage in hateful and spiteful matrimonial conflict.

What exactly does "**differences**" mean? Differences are conflicting opinions or actions stuck between spouses that concern behavior, traditions, principles, and approaches in relation to disagreement, marital style and role expectations. Differences can lead to conflict situations which consist of spoken and unspoken exchanges that reveal a clash of views or actions.

Marriage officially brings together a man and a woman; people from diverse households with differing environments, ways of existing and possibly even traditions and ethnicity. Seldom is there an instance of a perfect marriage. The nature or character of one spouse may be lovable and charming and the other terse or harsh. There *will* be clashes of interests and priorities.

When there is a clash, there is a need for honesty and a readiness to listen to diverse viewpoints for differences to build up the relationship and not cause resentment. In some cases it is suitable to give in to your spouse's viewpoints, and in other cases, your viewpoint must be spoken and supported, at least through "give and take."

Differences may change over time. Yet, with time, the way in which spouses cope with differences influences whether they help the marriage develop, or impede it to the point of ruin. In some cases, differences can be overlooked by a spouse and he/she can "let go" of their own viewpoint to take hold of the spouse's viewpoint.

I have found in years of praying with married couples who are facing differences that the emphasis with a wife is the need to be **heard and understood**. With husbands, the emphasis is more on being **open and understood**. I have heard spouses make statements like:

He doesn't understand what **I** *need . . .*
She didn't want to talk and **I** *did . . .*
He has not ever understood **my** *need*
I *need her to hear what* **I** *am saying*

Note the use of "I" and "my."

Differences can be resolved depending on our approach and attitude which leads to good or bad consequences. Both spouses must acknowledge that there is a need to be heard and respected for opinions in order for a relationship to be strong. Both spouses need to be receptive to how each other thinks and respect each other's viewpoint, or troubles may worsen.

Classic categories of differences perceived by married couples include expectations that are poles apart, conflicting opinions, personality characteristics (an outgoing personality versus a shy personality), and distinct values. Married couples must approach differences by understanding that some differences are not as significant, and it is acceptable to let the other spouse's view supersede your own in these situations. I have also discovered that some differences can transform into similarities through time and development of the marital relationship.

Certain differences are not major, but are causes of aggravation and irritation and having a positive attitude when dealing with them is required and good for the relationship. If differences are not spoken, resentment and anger can climax, causing differences to increase, grow and ruin the marital relationship. With some differences, it is okay to back off; but not with all differences because anger and bitterness may develop. I have found that if there is open-mindedness about each spouse's views, it can help cultivate a deeper and stronger relationship.

Let's explore some of the most counterproductive yet familiar ways husbands and wives handle differences and some keys that will open the door to resolution.

Fire First

This spouse usually has an extensive reputation of causing emotional and mental hurts and wounds, driving away the nearest and dearest of relatives and damaging the marriage to the point of divorce. Once this spouse is caught up in a quarrel or difference they fire at the outset, interrogating their spouse and raising questions afterward; if they ask questions at all.

The Key to Resolution: It is essential that the "Fire First" spouse learns how to listen and cease making impetuous choices and twisted decisions when it comes to having a dispute with their spouse. In Matthew 7:1–5 it states:

> *Do not judge and criticize and condemn others, so that you may not be judged and criticized and condemned yourselves. For just as you judge and criticize and condemn others, you will be judged and criticized and condemned, and in accordance with the measure you [use to] deal out to others, it will be dealt out again to you. Why do you stare from without at the very small particle that is in your brother's eye but do not become aware of and consider the beam of timber that is in your own eye? Or how can you say to your brother, Let me get the tiny particle out of your eye, when there is a beam of timber in your own eye? You hypocrite, first get the beam of timber out of your own eye, and then you will see clearly to take the tiny particle out of your brother's eye.*
>
> —AMP

This sort of spouse must look at their intentions and behavior instead of criticizing their spouse. The character flaws that perturb us in others are frequently the behaviors we hate in ourselves. If you are prepared to condemn your spouse, make sure you don't deserve similar criticism. Evaluate yourself first, and then forgive and help your spouse.

The Fan of Times Gone By

In the blink of an eye, he/she is clever enough to remember with precision, every blunder, slip-up and blooper made by their spouse. When a difference happens, "The Fan of Times Gone By" resorts to bearing a thorough catalog of their spouse's previous lapse in decision making and offenses.

The Key to Resolution: Let bygones be bygones. In Philippians 3:13, Paul says:

> *I do not consider, brethren, that I have captured and made it my own [yet]; but one thing I do [it is my one aspiration];* <u>forgetting what lies behind and straining forward to what lies ahead.</u>
> —AMP

Keep in mind that every one of us has done stuff for which we are sorry, and we all live in the dread of what we have been and, at the same instance, the faith of what we want to be. If your faith is in Christ and Christ is in your marriage, you can release what went before and look ahead to what God will help you and your spouse turn out to become.

The Quiet Combatant

This spouse grasps the motto from the past, "silence is golden," to an extreme scope. This spouse will not talk regardless of what you do until they get good and darn ready. In fact, recognizing that they are tormenting their spouse and making both their lives unhappy means absolutely nothing to these "Quiet Combatants."

The Key To Resolution: Such a spouse must stop being relationship combatants and pledge to being peacemakers.

> *Blessed (enjoying enviable happiness, spiritually prosperous—with life-joy and satisfaction in God's favor and salvation, regardless of their outward conditions) are the makers and maintainers of peace, for they shall be called the sons of God!*
> Matthew 5:9 (AMP)

The Cussin' Specialist

Once he/she senses a disagreement cropping up, this spouse lessens him or herself to name-calling, shouting a bombardment of hateful expressions and extremely explosive curse words. In his or her foul psyche, abusive words are the main technique to pass on their anger and disputes.

The Key To Resolution: This spouse must stop living to be hostile, become self-disciplined, and keep their tongue under control. Proverbs 13:3 states:

He who guards his mouth keeps his life, but he who opens wide his lips comes to ruin.

—AMP

As a spouse, if you have not mastered self-discipline, it can become fairly obvious in your choice of verbal communication. Words can devastate and tear down your spouse. Self-discipline begins with the language you choose when you are not in agreement with your spouse. Halt! Reflect prior to talking. As an alternative to being "The Cussin' Specialist," endeavor to have a controlled and kind tongue. Those with controlled and gentle words reflect before talking, recognize when silence is key, talk honestly while, simultaneously, looking for methods to encourage.

Did you land in any of these metaphors? If so, are you eager and ready to replace your behaviors? If you do not adjust these behaviors, you can virtually anticipate that your wedded days will be full of continued dissatisfaction and chaos.

Usually, men and women think, process and express thoughts and feelings differently. I need to talk issues out. I usually circle around the issue and end up repeating myself. I do not want my husband to solve the problem; I just want him to actively listen to me (as opposed to reading the paper or doing something else while I am talking).

On the other hand, Reggie must think things through first, and then he is ready to discuss his thoughts and sometimes, even his feelings with me. I cannot rush his process any more than he can rush my process. We respect each others differences and allow each other the time we need to work through issues.

We also value each other's opinions (most of the time) and seek each other's advice on issues. We have learned over the years that there is value in having someone you love and trust help you solve a problem or how you can examine a situation differently or from another perspective.

Most men can compartmentalize their feelings while most women cannot. That is why after you and your husband argue, he can have sex and you think he is crazy. He can tuck his feelings away, like putting files away in a drawer, and then deal with them later. Even if the argument was resolved, you still have to let your upset emotions settle.

Why would God make us so different? So, we must rely on communicating with each other and with God. If you do not learn how to discuss your feelings and thoughts with your spouse in a constructive way, you will never understand each other. And, if you do not pray and ask God how to relate to each other, those differences will cause a chasm between you, instead of drawing you closer together.

After much prayer, reading the Bible and several books, I realized that my perfectionism needed to be modified. God does not want your personality completely changed; He wants your personality under submission to Him. Being the oldest child, I loved being first, being right, being perfect. I had to learn that I need other people's advice and ideas, especially my husband's.

I also learned that my husband (or, anyone else) has his own way of doing things. There is no right or wrong way of doing everyday routine things. It is okay if he solves problems or tasks differently than I do. It may seem like a simple lesson but it was a process that took years. My husband and I had to listen to each other, pray and have patience as we worked this out.

Our house is still rather neat, the bed made in the morning, dinner dishes are still washed after eating (or, put in the dishwasher). However, the boots and shoes are not lined up perfectly by the door. Thank God! Nor, do I obsess over most things. Notice, I said: "most things." (I am still a work in progress.) My husband's laid-back attitude and don't-get-upset-over-everything has somewhat rubbed off on me and he has actually finished projects way before the deadline without my nagging!

My husband has told me how much he has learned from me regarding organization and finishing tasks in a timely manner. Furthermore, I have told him that he has taught me not to get so uptight about everything. As well as the fact that excellence is not perfection! An important lesson I have learned throughout the years.

I am so glad my husband is not like me. I have learned so much from him. He has helped me see that differences are a good thing. God loves when a husband and wife have different strengths so they can help each other. Enjoy your differences and learn from your husband as he learns from you.

If you think "differences" in your marriage take adjustments, let us dig deep into our souls for the next myth: Myth #7: " 'Submission' Is Optional for a Good Marriage."

Lay Bare Your Soul . . . Expose yourself to the truth!
"Behold, You desire truth in the inner being; make me therefore to know
wisdom in my inmost heart."
—Psalms 51:6

When you are faced with differences in your marriage, how do you handle yourself? What type of person do you become?

Did you find yourself in any of the metaphors in this chapter? If so, are you willing to change your behaviors?

How does your demeanor put a harmful rift between you and your spouse?

What might others say about the example they see in your marriage?

What might your children say?

Myth #7: "Submission" Is Optional for a Good Marriage

Four women are discussing submission and marriage . . .

Submission is based upon prehistoric, conservative, antiquated philosophies. This is the progressive age! You are archaic. How dare you talk about submission? Get with it, this is the twenty-first century!
—21-year-old single, never been married

I would get pleasure from submitting if my husband was picture perfect. But, he's not.
—44-year-old woman, married 5 years

Submission means the husband treats his wife like a slave. I don't think so!
—33-year-old divorcee

Submission will get in the way of my potential as a woman.
—27-year-old woman engaged to be married

As you can see, various opinions exist about submission in marriage. On the one hand are those who believe that the husband as head of the home has a delegated power from God over his wife. From this standpoint, the wife's reaction is submission. On the other side are those whose standard is the ultramodern equal marriage in which the partners are contemporaries in all matters. In the middle are scores of Christians who support a joint submission in love as the model, but also accept as true the husband having particular headship responsibilities. Then there are those who rebuff submission to a man and consider such submission as an Achilles' heel and limiting.

Being subject to another individual (also called submission) is an often misinterpreted concept. If you are like me, you were taught to be independent, speak up for yourself, and never be anyone's doormat. Then, we came to Christ and heard preachers speak about marriage; the first thing they would say is, "wives should be submissive to their husbands." The hair on the back of my neck would go up every time!

Why is the word "submission" so threatening? It is threatening because no one ever taught the **correct** Biblical meaning of submission. Essentially, we as women in the church have been trained, "women are to submit always and without qualification." Husbands and wives were never taught to revere and respect each other.

> Be subject to one another out of reverence for Christ (the Messiah, the Anointed One). Wives, be subject (be submissive and adapt yourselves) to your own husbands as [a service] to the Lord. For the husband is head of the wife as Christ is the Head of the church, Himself the Savior of [His] body. As the church is subject to Christ, so let wives also be subject in everything to their husbands. Husbands, love your wives, as Christ loved the church and gave Himself up for her, so that He might sanctify her, having cleansed her by the washing of water with the Word, that He might present the church to Himself in glorious splendor, without spot or wrinkle or any such things [that she might be holy and faultless]. Even so husbands should love their wives as [being in a sense] their own bodies. He who loves his own wife loves himself.
> —Ephesians 5:22–28 (AMP)

The Greek word for submission is **hupotasso** which means "to get under and lift up" or "to put in order." **Hupo** means "under" and **tasso** means "arrange" (as in Chain of Command). It does not mean obedience. "Submission" is also a military term referring to the equal sharing of tasks, to support, to fulfill one's part of the assignment. Every individual in an army is significant, but there is an arrangement to operate efficiently. (John Temple Bristow, *What Paul Really Said about Women,* pg. 47)

Submission is a voluntary arrangement of fitting under in a way that makes a complete whole. A wife who is loved by a husband who loves her as Christ loves the Church will not be afraid to submit—voluntarily fit—under her husband. Submission is not about control or who the boss is but about enjoying the leadership of a husband who is submitting to God and loving you as Christ loves the church.

Before you truly understand why submission to your husband is good for you and your marriage, let us first take a look at two reasons why wives bristle when they hear the word "submission":

1. present perspective on past hurts;
2. false expectations.

Present Perspective on Past Hurts

If you had lived in a bubble all your life or on a desert island, you may have never experienced any past hurts. Since we all live in the real world and experience and witness all kinds of relationships, we form our opinions and perspectives on relationships very early in life. Every negative or positive experience in our relationships form indelible imprints upon our hearts that shape our perspectives. These imprints, no doubt, affect the way you respond to your husband. Based upon past relationships, ask yourself these questions:

Have you forgiven your father or father figure for ungodly leadership in your home growing up? Are you harboring resentments against past boyfriends or past ex-husbands? Without even realizing it, sometimes you believe your husband is going to lie to you, not be a good provider, or going to cheat on you because you experienced that in a former relationship or witnessed that behavior in your home as a child.

With this kind of perspective, you put up walls to protect yourself. You cannot submit to your husband's ideas or leadership because you cannot be absolutely sure that he is being truthful and will not run out on you leaving you with bills and babies. So, you withhold part of yourself. Part of you does not trust your husband. Part of you does not want to be completely dependent upon his leadership.

False Expectations

While dating and even on the honeymoon, I think many women develop false expectations about how easy and carefree marriage will be. While dating, he agrees to everything you want to do. Preparing the wedding, he consents to just about everything you want. On the honeymoon, things couldn't be rosier. However, you cannot stay on your honeymoon forever. Eventually, you and/or your husband will return to work, start raising a family, helping kids with homework, taking kids to soccer practice and music lessons, paying bills, dealing with relatives, doing ministry and well . . . you get the picture.

On the honeymoon, there are usually no stressors or outside people to interfere with your marital bliss. In the "real" world, you and your husband are going to have to make all kinds of decisions. Decisions about the children; what home to buy; what bills to acquire; how to pay off those bills. Even decisions about spiritual matters.

When I was first married, I had an unconscious expectation that everything should be done my way. I say "unconscious" because if anyone had asked me, I would *never* have said that I expected all decisions in our marriage to be my decisions. Of course not! I think we all use the words "give and take," "compromise," "joint" when referring to how we will respond to the decision-making process in our marriages. However, we usually harbor false expectations about submitting to our husbands. I know I did!

I am a very independent woman who in the early years of my marriage wanted to control any and every decision made in our home. It did not matter to me how insignificant the concern was, I usually wanted the final say on the subject. I did not realize until much trial and error and many arguments with my husband, that I had an issue with control! I did not learn until I sought the Lord that I needed to be more interdependent upon my husband. I will explain the difference between independence and interdependence in the next section.

Let us now examine two beliefs you will have to live by and exercise faithfully if you want a successful, joyous marriage:

1. Forgive the people from your past; and
2. Enjoy being submissive based on realistic expectations of your husband.

Forgive the People from Your Past

You hear that and you know it to be true. How many messages have you heard preached on forgiveness? How many workshops at women's conferences have you attended where you wrote the person's name you must forgive on a piece of paper and after prayer tore up the paper as an act of "letting go"?

Well, it is true that we must forgive the past in order to move forward in the present and future. Your husband is not your father or a past boyfriend or former husband. Talk with your husband and tell him about your feelings of being abandoned or rejected or disrespected in the past. Ask your husband's forgiveness for holding him accountable for other men's failures. Pray to God and ask Him to help you to truly forgive and move on.

Enjoy Being Submissive Based on Realistic Expectations of Your Husband

There are two things that are going to help you enjoy being submissive to your husband:

1. Trust in God
2. The difference between independence and interdependence

First of all, I have learned that we are not on our honeymoon, and that we must face real circumstances and make real decisions together. I have accepted the fact that we are no longer dating, so he will have an opinion on everything NOW! Submission means to put all of myself—understandings, knowledge, opinions and energies—at the disposal of my husband. This never means subjecting myself to abuse nor does it mean I mindlessly acquiesce to everything my husband suggests. I am never treated as worthless or inferior but my thoughts and opinions are important in the decisions reached in our family.

Let me share with you one experience I had when my husband did not ask my opinion but simply told me not to do something. Years ago, during the Christmas holiday season, I was going to the shopping mall by myself to do my final shopping. Our daughters were young so he was going to baby-sit.

I had the money for shopping (out of our little budget at that time). I was about to put on my coat when all of a sudden he says, "You shouldn't go shopping tonight." I was shocked. I asked him,

"Why?" All he could say was, "You must not go shopping tonight."

Years ago, there were fewer shopping malls in Rochester than there are today so I was going to shop at the most popular mall. However, I took off my coat and prepared the girls for bed. I hardly ever was up late enough to watch the eleven o'clock news but I was up that night. The biggest news story that night was how young men were hiding under cars in the shopping mall—the one where I had planned to shop—and slashing women's heels. When women fell down, the men would steal the women's handbags and packages and run away. Several women had minor cuts but several more women were cut severely! That was the mall where I was supposed to do my shopping! What would have happened to me if I had not submitted to my husband? Well, I am glad I was safe at home. And, I was glad I had submitted to my husband!

I have learned to appreciate that my husband will make mistakes and that I should not have these unrealistic expectations that he will get it right all of the time. Even though he is a praying man, and asks for my opinions, he is not going to always make the right decisions. And, that is okay!

I have learned that my deference to my husband is a duty owed to the Lord. A wife's submission is not as much to her husband, a man, as it is to God and His plan for marriage. So, I am trusting that God will help my husband and his decisions. My husband has never made a decision that was so irreparable since he has accepted the Lord as the head of his life. I believe that God is watching out for me and will not allow my husband to steer us off our course!

The other key is knowing the difference between being independent and interdependent. Accepting this difference has helped me understand submission to a much better degree. Webster's dictionary defines "independent" as "not requiring or relying on others; not subject to the control of others." Webster defines "inter" as "reciprocal; occurring between; shared by" and "dependent" is defined as "relying on another for support." (*Merriam-Webster's Collegiate Dictionary* 11th ed., 2005)

A husband and wife are to rely on each other, depend on each other for support, encouragement and decision-making. You must share with each other your thoughts, hopes, dreams, aspirations, dislikes about the marriage, and ways to improve. There must be reciprocity—a give and take—and a submission from both parties.

An example of how interdependence works in marriage can be explained by Kathy Holmgren, who is married to a former head coach of the Green Bay Packers:

> *The older I've gotten, I realize that each one of us, we have to find our own life. If he's happy in what he does, that makes for a better partner for me. And he feels the same way about me. So he's really very nice about giving me opportunities to enrich myself and to really do the kinds of things that I like to do. . . . It's real important for each one of us to have our own life, so that I don't depend on him for my happiness. I have to be happy on my own. But we really do like to spend time together, so it's not like we lead separate lives. Whenever we can be together, we would opt for that, because we really like each other.*
> Packer Plus Online, 12/97 Mike and Kathy Holmgren Marriage Profile.

No matter how much I try to practice interdependence, I must admit, God is still working on me. Sometimes, I must practice expressing my feelings and thoughts in love and not in the heat of the moment. It is usually better if I take a few hours to calm down and pray before I approach my husband in anger. When we were first married, with every confrontation I could be found yelling. My husband was usually quiet. I took his quietness as consent. He merely listened but did whatever he wanted to do. I had to learn to discuss an issue quietly with my husband. I learned that yelling only made me look foolish and did not solve a thing. I could not change my husband—only God! I had to speak my case as calmly as possible and let God do the rest. Men hate yelling and nagging wives! The Bible says, . . . *It is better to dwell in a corner of the housetop [on the flat oriental roof, exposed to all kinds of weather] than in a house shared with a nagging, quarrelsome, and faultfinding woman.* (Proverbs 21:9 AMP) Now, do I speak calmly all of the time? Not hardly. Sometimes I revert to my fleshly ways: stubborn, whining and wanting my way. Ladies, submission is a process. However, with God's help, we can do all things.

Submission does not mean becoming a doormat. Submission is a basic building block in the smooth functioning of any marriage. God designed submission in marital relationships to thwart disorder and confusion. It is critical that women grasp that submission is not resignation, alienation or apathy. It does not mean weakness. God formed all people in His image, and all have equal value. Submission is about shared dedication and collaboration.

God calls for submission among equals. He did not make the male superior; He made a way for the male and female to work jointly in marriage. Jesus Christ, while equal with God the Father, submitted to Him to complete the plan for salvation. Similarly, even though equal to man under God, the wife should submit to her husband for the sake of their marriage and family.

Submission among equals is submission by choice, not by coercion. We serve God in these relationships by voluntarily submitting to our spouses. Submission is seldom a dilemma in families where both spouses have a strong connection with Christ and where each is concerned for the happiness of the other.

At the beginning of the chapter, there were comments from four women on their perspective of submission in marriage. Has your thinking changed from the way any one of those women think? Do you want to trust that God will look out for you as you submit to your husband? Do you believe that God wants you to be more interdependent and less independent in your marriage? Submission also is appreciated and practical when there is open communication in a marriage as we will learn in the next chapter: Myth # 8: "We Will Never Argue."

Lay Bare Your Soul . . . Expose yourself to the truth!
"Behold, You desire truth in the inner being; make me therefore to know
wisdom in my inmost heart."
—Psalms 51:6

How do you view submission in your marriage?

_____
_____
_____
_____

Have you discussed submission with your husband to learn his views? Are your husband's views biblical? If not, how will that affect the way you respond to your husband?

_____
_____
_____
_____

Myth #8: We Will Never Argue

It takes two to speak the truth—one to speak, and another to hear.
—Henry David Thoreau

Without open, honest, loving communication, you will never know each other's needs, desires, goals and plans. You will never know each other. When we see a happily married couple smiling at each other and finishing each other's sentences, we tend to think that there exists some mysterious blend of the "right" two people having been blessed to find each other and marry.

Then, when we see an unhappy couple, we tend to think that those two people are simply "wrong" for each other. However, more often then not, marital relationships are strained, suffer for years and lead to divorce court as soon as the children leave the home when one or both partners do not communicate their needs and desires. There are numerous books on effective communication. Get some and practice, practice, practice.

Let's discuss a few keys to open communication. Unconditional love, expressing your feelings and thoughts in love and the ability to reach compromises are keys to effective communication.

Learn to ask questions and he will see if the idea is feasible or not. Say, "Honey, that's really interesting. Tell me more. Now, how will we pay for that? Are you interested in doing that now or a few years from now? What's your timeframe? What should we give up in order to do this?"

Doesn't that sound better than if you say, "That's a stupid idea!"

In our early years of marriage, I wanted to win but he wanted to win, too. In actuality, we both lost. However, we did not have the tools to communicate effectively so we could clearly see each other's side of the argument and reach an amicable solution.

Before anything else, it is important to dispel the myth that your spouse should always know what you are thinking. Learning to have effective communication in marriage is one of the most important aspects of marriage that a couple can work on. No matter how long you have been married, you have experienced communication miscues. Here is an example:

> A husband of ten years, who was a news reporter, told his wife weeks before a golf tournament that he would be gone all day covering the event. The golf tournament was on a Sunday, not a normal work day for the news reporter. The night before the golf tournament, his wife heard him planning to meet the Executive Director of the non-profit organization hosting the golf tournament at 8:00 A.M.
>
> What are you doing tomorrow?" the wife demanded as the husband hung up the cellular phone. (Translation: You had better not be working on a Sunday.)
>
> "I'll be at the golf tournament, most likely most of the day," the husband replied. (Translation: Certainly she remembers.)
>
> "Don't you think you should have let me know that you were going to be gone for a whole Sunday?" (Translation: You forgot to pass this little tidbit of information on to me yet again).
>
> "Didn't I tell you ABC Non-Profit organization was having this golf fundraiser and asked me to serve as the Master of Ceremonies?" (Translation: I expect you to remember these things.)
>
> "No, you didn't." (Translation: You're going to pay for this.")

"Okay, okay." (Translation: Danger! Danger!)

This example of a communication miscue can give rise to the anger emotion. Anger comes from unrealized, unmet goals and expectations we have set for ourselves or we have allowed others to establish for us. For example, you expect to have just as many long night talks as you had before you were married. Those talks are not happening—this is what is called an unmet expectation.

Unmet Expectations + Hurt = Anger

Now you are angry and strike out by yelling. In actuality, you are hurt. Anger is usually the first emotion we will express when there are buried emotions begging to be dealt with, for example, grief, hurt and/or rejection. More often than not, we deal with anger by being passive-aggressive—being angry but expressing it in a disguised way. Or, we let out our anger by procrastinating—delaying doing something for our husband. And, probably the most favorite unhealthy way to deal with anger is through sarcasm.

Anger is like a can of hair spray. No matter how hard you concentrate the spray on your hair, you get some in the air, on the mirror, and on other people. When we do not deal with those unmet expectations, anger will spray out onto innocent people—like our children or co-workers.

When angry, do not sin; do not ever let your wrath (your exasperation, your fury or indignation) last until the sun goes down.
—Ephesians 4:26 (AMP)

If ventilated recklessly, anger can hurt your husband and ruin your marriage. If bottled up inside, it can trigger both spouses to grow to be hostile and nasty which will lead to the destruction of the marriage. In this passage of scripture, Paul tells us to deal with our anger immediately in a way that builds the marriage relationship rather than destroying it.

If we harbor our anger, we will give Satan an opening to initiate a split in the marriage. Don't let a day end before you begin to work on healing your marriage.

Anger and yelling will occur in relationships and in the marriage relationship. However, we should not sin nor should we let days and days go by before communicating our needs. Your husband cannot read your mind. You must sit down with him and communicate your needs, your hurts, your pain and your desires.

Contrary to widespread belief, anger is natural and healthy because it is a human emotion. Anger, in reality, is a useful signal to help persons recognize that there is something that should be worked out or made right somewhere, by hook or by crook. Anger, if appropriately dealt with, can help correct a potential offense.

Strong marriages are characterized by kind, encouraging and open communication. We want to build each other up in our marriages, never run our spouse down.

Let no foul or polluting language, nor evil word nor unwholesome or worthless talk [ever] come out of your mouth, but only such [speech] as is good and beneficial to the spiritual progress of others, as is fitting to the need and the occasion, that it may be a blessing and give grace (God's favor) to those who hear it.
—Ephesians 4:29 (AMP)

There are three (3) important parts to the verse written by Paul:

1. If you don't have something good to say, don't say anything at all. Do you remember your mother or grandmother saying this to you?
2. We should consider the needs of the listener. Your

spouse has a different set of needs than you. You should therefore listen to consider how best to encourage and support your spouse.
3. The purpose of talking in the first place should be to benefit the listener.

Check your motives. If your motives are to hurt and dishearten your spouse, then continue to address him with insults, hatred and discouragement. If your aim is to build up and support your spouse, then speak words of encouragement, tenderness and admiration to him. Your spouse will see you as a tender individual and he will always want to be near you. He will like to listen to you speak, as your words will "be like honey" to him. (Psalms 119:103)

Paul advises us against harsh talking, nastiness, and improper use of anger, spats, cruel language, and rude attitudes towards others. Instead of acting that way, we should be forgiving, just as God has forgiven us. Act in love toward your spouse, just as God acted in love by sending His Son to die for our sins.

So choose properly how you will use your words. You have the potential to build up, or to tear down, just by the choices you make.

Here are a few steps I have followed that have helped me when I am angry:

1. Pray. The easy, humbling act of asking for help from the Lord relaxes the heart and makes communication easier. First, I pray and ask God why am I so angry? Did I bring it on myself? Did I have a false expectation that my husband would do or say something but when he did not respond was I hurt? Did he even know what I expected?
2. Verbal Communication. Determine a time to dialogue. One of the most challenging difficulties when a couple is extremely active is finding the time to dialogue. Com-

munication takes a considerable amount of time. I calmly sit down with my husband and express my hurt, desire, need and/or expectations. Also, deal with anger without delay—not weeks, months, or even years later. Keep in mind, words spoken unwisely can't be taken back. Think, listen, and calm down before you respond.

3. Listening. Listen more carefully. Before moving on to talk about a resolution, make sure you truly grasp what your spouse is expressing. Many times the greatest anxiety with communication in a marriage comes from thinking that you are not being heard. By communicating and listening to my husband, I find out if he can or if he even wants to meet that particular need or desire of mine. Is it a realistic need that he can meet? If you want a date with your husband every week but he can only realistically agree to every other week and stick to it, then you should rejoice in reaching a compromise.

4. Concentrate on Values not Viewpoints. Real communication happens when we realize we need to concentrate on mutual values instead of differences in viewpoints. Generally we focus a quarrel on opposite viewpoints. (You reason Junior should be in bed by 7:00 P.M. and your spouse believes he should be in bed by 8:00 P.M.) As an alternative, concentrate on the fundamental values of the concern (kids should be well rested); they are almost the same for both spouses. Simply identifying mutual values makes talking about a resolution easier because you believe you are both on the same side.

When I have followed these steps, I have learned why I am angry and what to do about it. When I have not followed these steps, I end up yelling at my husband and must apologize later then follow these steps anyway.

Some couples have more serious anger issues that threaten

their safety. If that is your concern, you should seek professional help immediately. Here, I am discussing the normal frustrations that occur in marriages. If you do not know what is normal, talk with your pastor or a counselor. Seek marital counseling from competent, Christian professionals. Always get a referral from someone reliable.

How to Not Argue and Communicate Effectively

Here are **10 Communication Tools** I wish I had used in our early years of marriage:

1. **Ask:** If you can tell something is irritating your spouse, ask about it. Lots of times a husband wants to express his displeasure about the marriage, about his job, etc., but he doesn't want to come across as a grouch. Gradually draw it out from your spouse. Ask tenderly but candidly, "Is anything troubling you, Baby? I'd like to hear about it." Not only will you both feel better, but the dialogue may turn to deeper matters.

2. **Face-to-face:** Nothing substitutes for face-to-face discussions, but sometimes you may have to write a letter to your spouse. Try to select a time when you actually have time to talk and discuss issues out of earshot of the children and others. Hopefully, you have had time to pray first and collect your thoughts.

3. **Focus:** Focus on one problem at a time; not the whole bailiwick of them. See the problem as a challenge the both of you have; not just one of you.

4. **"I feel":** Try to always use "I feel" statements, instead of speech that sounds accusatory like "you always . . .", "you are . . .". By no means use declarations like "never" and "always." For example, "You never take the trash out." If you do, he will think of one time in 1956! Nor, "You are always late." He will

counter that too and you will have lost the meaning of what you were trying to say at the beginning.

5. **Laughter.** I have learned through the years that laughter between a couple can truly enhance a marriage. You must take time to play and laugh together. And, you must have your own "secret" jokes just between the two of you. You and your hubby will be in a public place and someone will say or do something that will jog your and your husband's memory about your "secret" joke and you both will laugh. For example, I coached one married woman whom I will call Sue as follows:

> Dr. C: What was your last "secret" joke just between you and your hubby?
>
> Sue: I apologized for not being more attentive to him a week ago and promised him a "brand new wife." So this week, I have really been so much better so I asked him at the end of the week, "do you see my 'newness' and he laughed."
>
> Dr. C: You go girl! Now, when he does something positive that you've been asking of him, say, "oh, I see the newness in you, too!" Keep the "newness" as a joke for a few more weeks. Then, at a "God-moment" you can expand on this "newness" theme into a more serious conversation about your and his feelings, dreams and desires.

Take laughter and turn it into a more in-depth intimate conversation that you long to have with your husband.

6. **Learn your husband's "love language":** One of my husband's "love languages" must be "service." When I cook, my husband is so turned on and he gets so excited. I, on the other hand, am turned on by "gifts" and "words of encouragement." Women complained in the focus groups I held that their husbands do not talk; do not communicate. Ladies, they are communicating. We just must learn to speak their languages. And, they need to learn our

languages. When your husband pays the bills on time, he is communicating love. When your husband insists that you wear your seatbelt in the car and lock your doors, he is communicating love. When he says, "sure, I'll baby-sit the children so you can go shopping," he is communicating love. Ladies, you must learn your husband's ways of communicating. Learn his love languages and encourage him to learn yours. Make it fun.

7. **Look for the signs:** Realize the painful reactions of your spouse may be a sign of hidden, past hurts (that you may or may not have contributed to). Don't insist that your way is the only way. Try to develop "another side" line of reasoning; trying to go beyond your side and his side and see "another side."

8. **"Nagging" is not synonymous with "communicating":** Proverbs 21:9 says, *It is better to dwell in a corner of the housetop [on the flat oriental roof, exposed to all kinds of weather] than in a house shared with a nagging, quarrelsome, and faultfinding woman.* The Bible does not say quarrelsome husband but wife! Interesting! Rather than nag my husband, I leave him notes. In other words, we have had a discussion and he agreed to do thus-and-so. My note is simply a reminder to him (not an "order" or "command").

9. **Shun insistence:** Don't insist that your way is the only way.

10. **Words do hurt:** Try to start the discussion with something he has done that was helpful, thoughtful and loving. In no way attack his character nor name call. The old saying, "sticks and stones may break my bones, but words will never hurt me" is a lie. Words do hurt. They sting. They wound. And, they cannot be taken back. Don't get caught up in name calling (Matthew 5:22). Name calling and bullying aren't Christ-like behaviors. They serve no purpose but to deliberately wound the other person. Don't give full vent to your anger. You may be upset at your spouse, but you don't have the right to allow your anger to run riot on him. Self-control is a fruit of the Spirit (Galatians 5:22–23). Cursing,

hitting, and breaking things aren't God-honoring behaviors. Yelling is not communicating. The past is nowhere as present as a yelling match with your husband. Harsh words cannot be taken back. They linger in your soul. When upset or angry, pray before having a discussion with your spouse.

Use these tools daily and pray daily asking God to strengthen you and your husband's communication together. Remember to compliment your husband when he does communicate.

The next chapter may not apply to every person who reads this book; however, in this day in age, as Christians, we must talk about the subject of divorce with Myth #9: "Love No Longer Lives Here."

Lay Bare Your Soul . . . Expose yourself to the truth!
"Behold, You desire truth in the inner being; make me therefore to know
wisdom in my inmost heart."

—Psalms 51:6

Are you angry with your spouse? Why?

_____
_____
_____
_____

What can you do to resolve your differences?

_____
_____
_____
_____

Are you grieving or pleasing God with your attitudes and actions?

_____
_____
_____
_____

Communication Prayer

Lord, help me to see all the things my husband does that communicates his love for me. Help me to communicate as a wise woman and not a foolish one. In the name of Jesus Christ, I am determined to take control of my tongue. My mouth shall utter truth. Help me not to nag nor be quarrelsome. Help me to play and joke more with my husband. Lord, help him to be the husband you want him to be. In Jesus' name I pray.
Amen.

Myth #9: Love No Longer Lives Here

Note for Reader: This chapter may not be for everyone, however, I believe it is extremely important to include. It is about the unspeakable "D" word—DIVORCE.

Redeemer is one of God's descriptions, and aren't we thankful! He loves us and gives us second chances in numerous areas—including marriage. Second marriages are by nature more complex and more susceptible for a second divorce than first marriages—over 60 percent divorce rate, compared to around 50 percent for first-time marriages.

The biblical model is marriage that lasts a lifetime. Christians sometimes must muddle through the splitting up of a marriage. Due to the fact that humans do not live up to the high ideals and standards of God, marriages do fold, flop or bomb. With the strong biblical emphasis on marriage as a lifetime commitment, divorce poses a heartfelt quandary for Christians.

The Bible teaches permanence as the standard; but sadly, human necks are yet stiff; and divorce for a variety of reasons still happens. The Gospels are filled with examples of how Jesus dealt with persons who were struggling with blame and disappointment, including one lady who had been married five times and who was living with a guy who was not her husband. When guiltiness was involved, Jesus did not diminish it; but in every case He acted to summon deliverance and freedom. Specifically, His purpose was not to criticize people but to help them start anew with God's mercy.

However, in many denominations and churches Christians do not want to deal with divorce. I found few Christian authors who wanted to tackle this sticky issue. I understand why. God hates divorce.

> "And this you do with double guilt; you cover the altar of the Lord with tears [shed by your unoffending wives, divorced by you that you might take heathen wives], and with [your own] weeping and crying out because the Lord does not regard your offering any more or accept it with favor at your hand. Yet you ask, Why does He reject it? Because the Lord was witness [to the covenant made at your marriage] between you and the wife of your youth, against whom you have dealt treacherously and to whom you were faithless. Yet she is your companion and the wife of your covenant [made by your marriage vows]. And did not God make [you and your wife] one [flesh]? Did not One make you and preserve your spirit alive? And why [did God make you two] one? Because He sought a godly offspring [from your union]. Therefore take heed to yourselves, and let no one deal treacherously and be faithless to the wife of his youth. For the Lord, God of Israel, says: I hate divorce and marital separation and him who covers his garment [his wife] with violence. Therefore keep a watch upon your spirit [that it may be controlled by My Spirit], that you deal not treacherously and faithlessly [with your marriage mate]."
> —Malachi 2:13–16 (AMP)

"Now when Jesus had finished saying these things, He left Galilee and went into the part of Judea that is beyond the Jordan; and great throngs accompanied Him, and he cured them there. And Pharisees came to Him and put Him to the test asking, Is it lawful and right to dismiss and repudiate and divorce one's wife for any and every cause? He replied, Have you never read that He Who made them from the beginning made them male and female, and said, For this reason a man shall leave his father and mother and shall be united firmly (joined inseparably) to his wife, and the two shall become one flesh? So they are no longer two, but one flesh. What therefore God has joined together, let not man put asunder (separate). They said to Him, Why then did Moses command [us] to give a certificate of divorce and thus to dismiss and repudiate a wife? He said to them, Because of the hardness (stubbornness and perversity) of your hearts Moses permitted you to dismiss and repudiate and divorce your wives; but from the beginning it has not been so (ordained). I say to you: whoever dismisses (repudiates, divorces) his wife, except for unchastity, and marries another commits adultery, and he who marries a divorced woman commits adultery."

—Matthew 19:1–9 (AMP)

In the book of Deuteronomy, Moses instituted some laws to help the victims of divorce. In the scripture from Malachi, men of the Old Testament were marrying heathen women who worshiped idols. Divorce was familiar, happening for no motive other than a yearning for change. This may sound familiar even in this day and age. Divorce in these times was practiced solely by men. They broke their commitment with their wives and disregarded the relationship involving a husband and a wife that God instills and his principle for them who love the Lord. Not only were men breaking their commitment with their wives, they were snubbing their noses at the bonding relationship and spiritual principle of being unified with God.

In the scripture from the book of Matthew, the Pharisees were trying to trick Jesus by having him choose sides in a theological controversy. Two main groups had two opposing views of divorce. One group supported divorce for almost any reason. The other believed divorce could be allowed only for marital unfaithfulness. However, in his answer, Jesus focused on marriage rather than divorce.

While Christian marriages should model God's love for His bride, the church, we are getting divorced almost as fast as married people who do not have Christ in their lives. A study released by The Barna Group, of Ventura, California, in September 2004 explains that the probability of married adults getting divorced is identical among born again Christians and those who are not born again.

Among all adults eighteen and older, three out of four (73 percent) have been married and half (51 percent) are currently married. Among those who have been married, more than one out of every three (35 percent) have also been divorced. One out of every five adults (18 percent) who have ever been divorced has been divorced multiple times.

Born again Christians have the same possibility of divorce as do non-Christians. Among married born again Christians, 35 percent have experienced a divorce. That figure is equal to the outcome among married adults who are not born again: 35 percent. Multiple divorces are also surprisingly customary among born again Christians. Barna's figures show that nearly one-quarter of the married born agains (23 percent) get divorced two or more times.

In questioning the Christian married women in my focus groups in preparation for this book, I found that about half of these women were divorced at least once and a few divorced twice. Some did not have Christ in their lives when they were married the first time. Some divorced because their husbands were physically abusive. True love cannot exist if one's self-esteem is emaciated. And, in some cases the women divorced because they felt their self-esteem was being denigrated constantly whether through physical, verbal or emotional abuse. And, in some cases—all three. I do not believe that God wants you to be in a marriage where someone is beating you and making you fear for your life (and sometimes, for the lives of your children).

Whatever your reason for your past divorce, if you are a Christian now, then forget the things of your past as it says in Philippians 3:13–14 (NKJV):

Brethren, I do not count myself to have apprehended; but one thing

I do, forgetting those things which are behind and reaching forward to those things which are ahead, I press toward the goal for the prize of the upward call of God in Christ Jesus.

Are you having a difficult time forgetting the things that happened in your rocky, maybe tumultuous marriage? You are not alone! Here is a letter from a newly divorced woman:

Dear Dr. Cynthia,

    I am a Christian woman age thirty and newly divorced. We have one small son age three. My ex-husband and I were married for seven years before he came home one day from work and asked for a divorce. I was shocked! I did not see it coming! We had very few problems and everything seemed to be okay. We both worked a lot of hours to pay bills we both accumulated before marriage (including college loans). And, our sex life was almost non-existent but he seemed okay. He never complained. We were both tired. He loves our son and is a wonderful father. I thought he loved me however, he said he likes me but is no longer in love with me. I am devastated! How could this have happened after seven years of marriage?

Sincerely,
Devastated

Dear Devastated,

    I can only imagine how distraught you must be right now. I am so sorry. One never marries thinking they will have a child then be divorced and a single parent. You, of course, are asking "Why me?" You are wrestling with all the answers that pop in your head. Listen to this . . .

And Jacob was left alone; and there wrestled man with him until the breaking of the day.

—Genesis 32:24

Like Jacob, you and your son were left alone. You are disillusioned and devastated to discover that your husband abandoned you because he no longer loved you. That is painful! He stood at the altar before God and the witnesses and vowed to love you until death do you part. You probably feel as if he has died (or, sometimes you wish he had because you are so angry). This is all understandable. Feel the pain and anger (***really*** feel it) but do not get stuck there and become bitter. Seek God even more. You will learn that you can survive the loss of your husband but you cannot survive without your Lord and personal Savior, Jesus Christ. He, alone, can help you overcome your loss, pain and anger.

You did not indicate whether you went to counseling so I will assume you did not. Counseling may have helped but, of course, both must be willing to go and to save the marriage. You can no longer beat yourself up with "maybes," "ifs" and "buts." However, there were red flags flying high as warning signs that your marriage was in trouble. I would recommend that you go to a reputable, Christian counselor to help you recognize those warning signs and resolve your feelings so you do not carry that bitterness nor misunderstandings into another marriage.

Even though I have never experienced a divorce, I do know that God wants you free from past hurts and pains (physical, emotional and spiritual). He wants you to live an abundant life (John 10:10). And, I know without a shadow of a doubt—as you must know and believe with your whole heart—that "there is therefore now no condemnation to those who are in Christ Jesus, who do not walk according to the flesh, but according to the Spirit." (Romans 8:1 NKJV)

You must not allow anyone to condemn you for being a divorced woman. Christ does not condemn you so why should you allow others? Stop listening to Satan's lies and move on with your life. Love can live in your home and heart once again. True love. The kind of love God ordains for His children. However, first, before you even think about marrying again, consider these questions:

1. Are you healed emotionally?
2. Are you still blaming yourself for the divorce?
3. Are you still blaming your ex-husband for the divorce?
4. Are you angry with anyone? Are you angry with God?
5. Have you forgiven yourself? Have you forgiven your ex-husband?

You probably understood why I asked questions #1–4, but do you understand why I asked question #5? You must (there is no way around it) forgive yourself and your ex-husband. Forgive yourself for thinking you should never have married him. And, forgive him because God commands it. Read Matthew 6:14–15 and Matthew 18:21–35:

> For if you forgive people their trespasses [their reckless and willful sins, leaving them, letting them go, and giving up resentment], your heavenly Father will also forgive you. But if you do not forgive others their trespasses [their reckless and willful sins, leaving them, letting them go, and giving up resentment], neither will your Father forgive you your trespasses.
> —Matthew 6:14–15 (AMP)

Then Peter came up to Him and said, Lord, how many times may my brother sin against me and I forgive him and let it go? [As many as] up to seven times? Jesus answered him, I tell you, not up to seven times, but seventy times seven! Therefore the kingdom of heaven is like a human king who wished to settle accounts with his attendants. When he began the accounting, one was brought to him who owed him 10,000 talents [probably about $10,000,000], and because he could not pay, his master ordered him to be sold, with his wife and his children and everything that he possessed, and payment to be made. So the attendant fell on his knees, begging him, Have patience with me and I will pay you everything. And his master's heart was moved with compassion, and he released him and forgave him [canceling] the debt. But that same attendant, as he went out, found one of his fellow attendants who owed him a hundred denarii [about twenty dollars]; and he caught him by the throat and said, Pay what you owe! So his fellow attendant fell down and begged him earnestly, Give me time, and I will pay you all! But he was unwilling, and he went out and had him put in prison till he should pay the debt. When his fellow attendants saw what had happened, they were greatly distressed, and they went and told everything that had taken place to their master. Then his master called him and said to him, You contemptible and wicked attendant! I forgave and cancelled all that [great] debt of yours because you begged me to. And should you not have had pity and mercy on your fellow attendant, as I had pity and mercy on you? And in wrath his master turned him over to the torturers (the jailers), till he should pay all that he owed. So also My heavenly Father will deal with every one of you if you do not freely forgive your brother from your heart his offenses.

—Matthew 18:21–35 (AMP)

In these New Testament scriptures, Jesus Christ gives a shocking word of warning about forgiveness: if we refuse to forgive others, God will also refuse to forgive us. Whenever we ask God to forgive us for sin, we should ask ourselves, "Have I forgiven the individuals who have offended, persecuted or mistreated me?"

There are many other scriptures on forgiveness that you could read but definitely start with these. If you are feeling tortured in your soul (mind, will and emotions), you clearly need to read Matthew 18:21–35 over and over again. If you are holding on to unforgiveness, you will be tortured day and night until you release and forgive. Unforgiveness is a poison that will cause you to become a bitter woman as well as sick in your body.

The divorced women in our focus groups were all remarried to Christian men and could seek their understanding of their past hurts. However, if you need counseling from your pastor or a competent professional, do not hesitate to seek it out. Take time to resolve your first marriage through prayer, therapy, and pastoral care. God is the mighty Counselor and can heal you, if you will only bring your hurts to Him. For some of us, we need a counselor to walk us through the steps to freedom. Divorce can be a hot and divisive topic both in Scripture and in churches, and must be well thought-out on a case-by-case basis to determine the sort of pastoral care required for healing.

If you are contemplating re-marriage or are already in a second (or third, or fourth) marriage, the best assistance I can give you is to be frank with your soon-to-be (or already-is) spouse, take time together with your spouse and discuss expectations. Discuss the unique styles you each bring to the re-marriage and discuss compromises. Pay attention to your spouse and have compassion.

Frequent "connection time," focusing just on the marital relationship and having fun, is necessary for a victorious remarriage. Grace and Stan have four children between them. Stan has one daughter, age ten, and Grace has one son, age five. When asked when the last time they had an exclusive "connection time" was, Grace froze and Stan became stiff. "Too long to recall," Stan admits. Remarriages with children especially need "connection time." This may demand pulling back on time with friends and relatives, church work, and other responsibilities. Children take a lot of time, so your "connection time" must be protected and preserved.

Both you and your spouse bring strong thoughts from your prior relationships about what you do and do not want to be like as a spouse and what you want your spouse to be like. It is not your spouse's responsibility to make up for your ex-spouse's mistakes. It is both your and your spouse's duty to pinpoint and share your expectations of yourself and your spouse and discuss any differences.

Keep in mind that marriages, and remarriages, are a "labor of love." It is not just how much you love your spouse and your spouse loves you, but how the two of you communicate and deal with conflicts and disagreements. Even though troubles and tribulations will most indubitably develop, it is crucial to consider that remarriages need the same valuable and regular encouragement and cultivation as first marriages.

Unlike television shows, second marriages aren't fail-safe. Remarriages need the same dedicated and constant development as first marriages. No matter what your juncture in life or situation, with some additional attention and real interaction, your second marriage can be successful.

We now recognize that marriage, whether it is #1 or #2, is a "labor of love," but, in marriage there is also "sweet sex"! Last, but absolutely not least, let us devote some time to Myth #10: "Sex Is Love."

Lay Bare Your Soul . . . Expose yourself to the truth!
"Behold, You desire truth in the inner being; make me therefore to know
wisdom in my inmost heart."
—Psalms 51:6

Memorize Romans 8:1, John 10:10, Philippinas 3:13–14 and any other scriptures that will speak TRUTH to you.

Adults may lament the loss of a prior marriage, the demise of the "love" dream, the loss involved by changes that materialize because of divorce. Have you mourned your loss?

_____
_____
_____
_____

Studies have revealed that most people do not have exceptionally upbeat thoughts toward an ex-spouse. When couples make an effort to ease conflicts concerning ex-spouses, it enhances the marital value of the remarriage. Have you dealt positively with your previous relationship?

_____
_____
_____
_____

Countless remarriages include children. Getting used to stepchildren can take time. Relationships with new stepchildren are just forming and should not be hurried. Have you accepted the changes in the structure of your family unit?

_____
_____
_____
_____

Myth #10: Sex Is Love

Affection. Romance. Sex. Love. We often interchange these words. Consciously, we know each word has a different meaning but subconsciously we go through life in our marriage interchanging the true meaning of these extremely important words which evoke powerful emotions.

You'd never recognize by paying attention to the expressions in the current culture nowadays that sex was God's design, but it's true. He intended it not only as a way for reproduction, but also to be enjoyable and intensely fulfilling. Regrettably, many of us have shaped our opinions about sex from the society around us instead of from God's standpoint.

Your heart will be broken by your second year of marriage if you do not understand the true meaning behind each emotionally laden word. When you take a vow on your wedding day to love your husband until death do you part, what are you really expecting from him?

You, like most wives, are expecting love, romance, affection and sex—and quite often. You may not understand your husband's deep need for sex anymore than he understands your need for affection, states Dr. Willard F. Harley Jr. in his book, *His Needs Her Needs*.

Affection and Romance

Women crave affection and romance from their husbands. *Webster's Dictionary* defines affection as *"fond or tender feeling; warm liking: usually distinguished from love."* Romance is defined as *"to be fanciful or imaginative in thinking and talking; court; woo."* Why does it seem that some men know how to "court," and "woo" and "be imaginative" while they are dating but as soon as they say "I do," the romance and affection seem to decrease as the years pass away?

One of the main complaints wives have about their husbands in our Marriage Retreats is that their husbands no longer court them, woo them, show affection except on special occasions (for example, Valentine's Day). Husbands, your wives crave romance and affection. They need it like they need air! Wives, you can beg, plead, cry and nag your husband for more romance and affection but you will only become frustrated and angry. And, he will be exasperated and probably give up even trying.

My recommendation to wives is to "sow what you want to reap." Demonstrate to him what you want and need. If you like holding hands, take his hand. If you like back rubs, rub his back. If you want love notes left for you, leave them for him. If you want a cup of coffee in bed, bring him a cup in bed. Then water your planting with prayers. Ladies, your husbands will reciprocate! It is a biblical principle that God will fulfill.

We all want our husbands to whisper romantic, sexy words to us like King Solomon did to his bride in Song of Solomon. Ladies, you may have to teach him what you want. You cannot argue what you want or cry about it; teach him by example. Romance is setting out a negligee on a neatly made-up bed. Romance is a phone call to your husband in the middle of the day and whispering something sexy to him over the phone. Romance is leaving him an affectionate note beside his car keys before he goes to work. Romance is touching him and saying how much you appreciate him.

I loved the song by Bishop T.D. Jakes, "You are My Ministry." Wives, we must learn to minister to our husbands. We must learn to put them ahead of girlfriends, shopping malls, television, church work, even our children. We get caught up in our own desires and wants and forget that we should be providing a safe haven for our husbands; providing an atmosphere that promotes trust, communication, love and respect. Yes, our husbands have responsibilities too, but this book is for women!

When I learned to die to self, study my husband, ask him what his needs were and how could I fulfill them, my husband was more affectionate and more romantic. Even better and more fulfilling than the "courting" days. Wives, you cannot be afraid to communicate your needs in a calm manner. Communication is key for every area of your marriage.

What does all of this have to do with "sex"? Plenty! When the husband is meeting his wife's needs and she is meeting his needs, sex will be intimate, healing and as loving as God intended. Sex is not just for procreation but for the pleasure and happiness for both the husband and wife.

Wives, how do you become your husband's lover?

1. Ask him what he likes and dislikes.
2. Be your husband's lover! Studies show that men respond to sight. So, wives, wear sexy lingerie often; undress naked in front of him, do a "strip tease" number in the privacy of your bedroom for him. Ladies, stop feeling self-conscious of your size or shape; he is probably not the size or shape when you first married him either. Be your husband's "mistress" in the bedroom. I know it's hard sometimes to feel sexy and be sexy after a hard day at work, chauffeuring the children all over town, doing laundry, and the list goes on, but every now and then you need to "surprise" him with an erotic dance with whipped cream on his pecs (that you lick off).

3. Give him a suggestive wink.
4. Rub his leg under the table.
5. Pamper him and fuss over him.
6. Believe the best about him.
7. Be his #1 cheerleader and encourager.
8. Speak truth in love, calmness and honesty.
9. Be appreciative when he does do something you like.
10. Maintain a prayer life and church attendance.
11. Try to see things from his perspective sometimes; not just your own.
12. Have a candlelight dinner ready for him from time to time.
13. Set up a picnic in the living room.
14. Hold him, hug him and reassure him when he is hurt or burdened or discouraged.
15. Give him your undivided attention when he wants to talk.

Wives, it is important for you to understand that for most men, they cannot separate sex from love. Your husband's self-esteem is tied very closely with being desirable by you. If you do not tell and show your husband that you truly desire him sexually, his self-esteem suffers. Your husband needs sexual fulfillment in order to respond emotionally. And, you need emotional fulfillment in order to respond sexually. Yes, men and women are so different on many different levels. And, the sooner we learn this, the better off we will be in our marriages.

Wives and husbands may argue about closeness, intimacy, and affection. Wives want more hand-holding, touching, kissing and loving words when not having sex. Pause for a moment: reflect on the tone of the household in which your husband was raised. He may have been raised in an unemotional household while you were raised in a household where hugs, kisses and "I love you" were the order of the day. Trust me, God can change him! Your husband may not come all the way over to your intimate way of showing affection however; God can bring him to a happy middle. I am a witness!

People see my husband now—holding my hand, kissing me, teasing me affectionately but they should have seen us thirty-six years ago. Do not get me wrong, my husband has always loved me, respected me, and was affectionate in *his* way however, I wanted more. With much prayer, discussions with my hubby and sowing seeds of what I wanted to reap, I am happy to say, he has gone past mid-ground and is giving me more and more of what I so desire. Why? He knows that as a God-fearing, God-loving husband, he wants—with all his heart—to please me. WOW! Did it happen overnight? No. However, I had to pray, be patient, communicate my needs to my hubby, and sow the seeds of affection and romance that I wanted to reap.

Love

When we stand at the altar on our wedding day in front of God and witnesses and vow to love each other until death do us part, have you actually thought that you are promising to fulfill I Corinthians 13:4–8a (AMP):

> Love endures long and is patient and kind; love never is envious nor boils over with jealousy, is not boastful or vainglorious, does not display itself haughtily. It is not conceited (arrogant and inflated with pride); it is not rude (unmannerly) and does not act unbecomingly. Love (God's love in us) does not insist on its own rights or its own way, for it is not self-seeking; it is not touchy or fretful or resentful; it takes no account of the evil done to it [it pays no attention to a suffered wrong]. It does not rejoice at injustice and unrighteousness, but rejoices when right and truth prevail. Love bears up under anything and everything that comes, is ever ready to believe the best of every person, its hopes are fadeless un-

der all circumstances, and it endures everything [without weakening]. Love never fails [never fades out or becomes obsolete or comes to an end].

In order for love to truly flourish in your marriage, you must understand and fully practice God's definition of love as found in I Corinthians 13. Our love must be patient and kind; not self-seeking; not envious; never easily angered; not keeping long mental lists of each and every wrong.

When I coach married couples and tell them that love is ***selfless,*** they look at me with that glazed look in their eyes as if to say, "If I try to be selfless he (or she) will walk all over me, and you know, Mama didn't raise no fool!" The I Corinthian 13 type of love is a strong love—not wimpy—and definitely not a doormat kind of love. It is a love filled with mutual respect, a willingness to learn what satisfies or annoys each other, an understanding of true compromise, an appreciation of even the small things done for each other, an insatiable need to learn what makes my spouse tick.

Love is ***expressed*** when you say: "Oh that was the best sex." "Thanks for the beautiful flowers." "I'm so enjoying our day together with no children and no phones." What we are ***actually*** saying is: you are being so selfless and considering my feelings. What would happen if we each considered the other's feelings and emotional needs before we said or did anything?

Most women equate love as more of an emotional or physical need (romance or affection). If your husband sucked your toes for an hour, that would be love for some women. However, that is not how most men show love. Men show love by paying the bills (or providing his paycheck so you can pay the bills) and by doing "things."

When my husband goes out in the morning to get me coffee from Dunkin' Donuts, kisses me and then goes out again to go to his destination, he is showing me love. When he gets the toilet fixed (and I only have to remind him once), he is showing me love.

(Even though he uses the toilet too, but in his mind, he is showing *me* love.)

When he takes my car to get "gassed up" (without me even having to ask), he is expressing love. When Reginald nags me about wearing my car seatbelt, he is showing his love for me. Ladies, I know, it is not sexy or exciting but it is how most men express love.

Sexual Intimacy

Sexual union is first and foremost a means of communication. We communicate powerful messages to each other and to the Lord when we join ourselves sexually. It is our most intimate form of communication, enabling us to say things about our spiritual oneness that words cannot.
—Christopher & Rachel McCluskey, *When Two Become One Enhancing Sexual Intimacy in Marriage,* Revell, Grand Rapids Michigan, 2004. pg. 38

Before we discuss sexual intimacy, let us begin with the topic of touching—physically, emotionally and spiritually. Touching is a much overlooked, underutilized demonstration of love and affection in a marriage. We are so busy taking care of children, working, volunteering in church and in the community that we forget to touch our husbands (unless we are having sexual intercourse). Sex is desire. Touching is need. How often do you and your husband touch each other every day? Touching each other should be a normal, everyday sign of affection. It should not be just a signal for sex. Touch his arm, his cheek; rub his back as you pass by him. Touching demonstrates intimacy; shows him you care just for him; lets him know you are thinking about him. You should not just touch your husband physically but you should touch him emotionally. Emotional touching involves your eyes, your voice, and your smile. Show tenderness to your husband. Life is difficult and offers many challenges so be tender to your spouse. Not always nagging and telling him to take out the trash, walk the dog, fix the toilet, punish little Johnnie, and on and on.

Touching spiritually is a deeper level of intimacy. Are you praying for your husband? Does your relationship with your spouse reflect the relationship you have with the Lord? I learned that in order to have a deep relationship with Reginald that I must pray and be intimate with the Lord. It is in my relationship with God that I learn to have a deeper relationship with my husband.

Sex should be more than "slam, bam, thank you ma'am." Sex should be a pleasurable experience for both of you. Sex should be fun, adventurous, exciting, and breathtaking—at least most times. You should feel fireworks going off in your inner core radiating from the top of your head to the bottom of your toes—at least most times. You should have sexual intercourse as often as you both want it—at least most times. If you are not experiencing what I have just mentioned (or, something similar), then we need to talk, my sister-girl!

Why did I say "at least most times"? Life happens. We do not live a fairy tale life. Children deplete our energy. Illnesses come. Lives are hectic. And, the first thing that often suffers is your sexual intimacy with your spouse. Just like you must take the time for honest, open communication with your spouse, you will have to take time to enjoy each other sexually. When your children are young, this is even more important. Babies and young children will occupy almost every waking moment. As unromantic as this sounds, you may have to schedule those sexual escapades, especially if you are busy people.

You think you had great sex in the very beginning of your marriage; well let me tell you, sex gets better over time. Sex gets better over time, if you both have invested time. Time to communicate what turns each of you on or off. Moments to explore areas on each other's body that screams with erotic joy; to know how you best achieve an orgasm; time through the years to create wonderful memories of laughter, joy and intimacy.

Sex is extremely important in a marriage. However, communication, patience, practice and desire are the keys to unlock the door of sexual passion and pleasurable intercourse. But what happens when sex stops suddenly between you and your husband. Read this letter and my response, please.

Help Dr. C!

My husband will not have sex with me! I am thirty-two and he is thirty-six. We have not had sex in over two months. My husband and I dated for a year. We both had been saved for quite a few years and were celibate the whole while we were dating and engaged. When we got married, we had sex ALL THE TIME! We could do it anytime, anywhere. We just wanted to give each other pleasure.

After about two years of marriage I cannot even sweet-talk him into the mood. (I am in great shape by the way.) Before I forget, I know he is not seeing anyone else. He had that happen in his parents' marriage and he has talked about the profound psychological and emotional wounds that happen.

My husband is also not extremely demonstrative with his affection. I am forever asking him to hug me or hold me. I detest having to ask him because I feel like he is a machine just doing what I want him to do. I don't think this situation is fair and I get angry at him. I have no outlet but divorce.

HELP!

Sexless Scarlet

Dear Sexless Scarlet:

I know you are disheartened, frustrated, upset, angry and ready to head to divorce court. I truly understand. Before you go the route of a divorce, take a deep breath and let us pause to pray. You will need the wisdom of the Lord to help you navigate these rough waters.

Make your request known to God through this prayer:

Lord, open my understanding to my husband's and my lack of sexual intimacy. Soften my heart because it is hardening and closing toward my husband. Lord, help me not to be angry because anger is blinding me. Lord, I need wisdom for you said in your Word in James 1:5, "if any of you lacks wisdom, let him ask of God, who gives to all liberally and without reproach, and it will be given to him." Work in me Lord, as you also work in my husband to solve this issue to your glory. In Jesus' name, I pray and believe. Amen.

Now, ask yourself these questions:

1. Is my husband under unusual stress on his job? Is he afraid of being laid-off or fired?
2. Is he worried about any family situations? Are his parents or close siblings ill?
3. How are you and he doing financially?

If your husband is worried about any of the above for the last two months, then emotionally he could be detached and too distraught for sexual intercourse. If you believe the answers to all the above questions are "no," then ask yourself these questions:

1. Has my husband lost or gained weight in the past two months?
2. Has his pattern of eating or sleeping changed?
3. Is he lethargic, high strung or otherwise emotionally different?

If the answer is "yes" to any of these questions, your husband needs to see a medical doctor immediately. He could be depressed, have diabetes, high blood pressure or some other medical condition that needs to be treated right away. And, whether men want to admit it or not, their hormones get "out of whack" in middle-age just like ours do.

Because men typically do not go to the doctor for complete physicals, it is probably a good idea for your husband (and you) to have a complete (I do mean complete) physical and blood work-up.

Here is another question to ponder: Have you both decided to start trying to get pregnant and now he has changed his mind without telling you? You did not mention that in your letter but I thought I would ask. PLEASE do not try to get pregnant *now*, until you both resolve this issue *completely*.

I was saving this set of questions for last because these are probably the more difficult ones to answer and then deal with as God would have us:

1. Is your husband involved in gambling, pornography or drugs of any kind?
2. Or, is he reliving past sexual abuse that he suffered as a child?

As you can see, there could be any number of issues that your husband could be dealing with—alone. Christian counseling could be just what he needs. Of course, convincing him to go can be another matter entirely. I suggest you and he plan a dinner date at a nice restaurant. Just the two of you. Wear his favorite dress and fix your hair and make-up just the way he likes it. Then toward the end of dinner say something like this:

"Honey, my self-esteem is hitting rock bottom. I need help. We no longer have sex or any kind of intimacy, like hugging or cuddling unless I ask you. That hurts me because I am feeling unloved and undesirable. [Keep the message in "I" terms.] All I can think about is how we used to be: We had sex all the time and we enjoyed each other so much. Honey, please tell me what you are feeling right now? What can I do to help us? Can we please go talk to someone? A doctor? Our Pastor? A counselor?"

Sexless Scarlet, I know you are frustrated and angry and rightfully so. But, if you would heed my last bit of advice as well, I believe God will allow you and your husband to have a victorious testimony. As you know, you did not get married to get a divorce. You must TRUST God in every situation.

Please give your marriage more time. Please give your husband more time. Now, here is my last bit of advice. For the next month, just be soft, kind, and sweet to him and do not mention having sex, hugging or anything that is intimate. Stroke his ego, tell him how much you love and appreciate him. Pray and Fast. I believe God will turn this situation around and you will have magnificent sex with him again.

I know that Sexless Scarlet's concerns are a reality in many Christian marriages. This is just one of many complaints I hear from Christian and non-Christian women. After counseling married women for years and listening to them in our focus groups in preparation for this book, I learned there are also numerous myths floating around about sex. Let us discuss a few of them.

"Do Not Kick Off Sex" Myth

As a Christian wife, I felt I could not initiate sex with my husband. Somehow I thought that was not being holy.

Sex inside marriage is ordained by God and therefore holy. The key here is not whether the wife is holy if she initiates sex but why she does not feel holy if she does "kick it off." Have you been told that "good girls" do not make the first move? Do you equate sex with something dirty? Sex is not dirty no matter who initiates it—the wife or the husband.

This fear is from the devil and must be discussed with your husband. Have you and your husband prayed about this fear? Ask your husband does he want you to make the first move sometimes. You may be surprised when he says an exuberant, YES! Remember, *"For God did not give us a spirit of timidity (of cowardice, of craven and cringing and fawning fear), but [He has given us a spirit] of power and of love and of calm and well-balanced mind and discipline and self-control."* (II Timothy 1:7 AMP)

If you were sexually abused as a child or teen, you may need to seek counseling from a competent, professional God-fearing counselor. Have your husband go with you. You must and can face this together. God wants you free to enjoy *all* the benefits of marriage.

"Sex and Intimacy Fade with Age" Myth

The older you get, the less you want to have sex.

Now, to the myth that sex and intimacy fade with age. Ladies, do not let it! With hormonal changes constantly occurring in our bodies (premenstrual syndrome, pregnancies, postpartum moods, perimenopause), sometimes women just aren't in the mood. Men's bodies go through changes too but again, this book is for and about us women. Even when you may not be in the mood for sexual intercourse or your body is not cooperating with you, you can always be intimate with your husband. Lay naked together and just hold one another. Cuddle together on the sofa and watch a movie together.

If you are experiencing long periods of not desiring sex, go see your doctor; it could be physical. As you age, your vagina may become dry and tight. There are many over the counter products, like K-Y Jelly, to use which work beautifully. And, always talk to your husband about your feelings.

And another thing! When women are no longer in their child-bearing years, they feel less stress about becoming pregnant. Also, women are not as tired from caring for babies and toddlers. As teens move out of the home, wives have more time and more freedom to be less inhibited and more energy to truly show their hubby that sex is still important.

Illnesses are always a factor, as we grow older. However, as I grow older, I am learning the importance of eating healthy, exercising, getting adequate sleep, visiting the gynecologist, avoiding so many sweets, etc. In doing all of this, I have more energy, feel better about myself and am quite eager to enjoy my husband sexually.

Sex with your spouse never has to grow stale, old nor routine. Nor does it have to lessen, as you grow older.

"Boring Sex" Myth

Sex will get boring after a while with the same man.

Why should it? If you and your hubby have sex the same night or nights each week, the same time and in the same positions, I guess sex might get boring. Try these tips instead:

1. Set your alarm and have sex in the early morning hours instead of late at night.
2. Have sex in a different room of your house.
3. Try other sexual positions.
4. Be sure to discuss what you each like and dislike sexually (**not** during intercourse but during a different time when you are both relaxed).
5. Wear sexy lingerie and do a strip tease for him.
6. Massage each other before the sexual act.
7. Be creative!
8. Pray and ask God for ideas!

"Sex Is About Size and I Am Too Fat Now" Myth

I have gained about thirty pounds since we were first married. I no longer feel sexy so I usually do not even want to have sex.

Study the paintings of the master artists and you will find beautiful, plus-size women. Sexuality is less about your size, and more about your self-confidence. Please do not fall into the Hollywood stereotype of what a woman should look like. Remember, your husband may not look exactly the same as when you married him either.

Your husband wants you to "want him" and you must feel self-confident to express that in a sexual manner. I went through those same self-doubts myself. I, too, am not the same smaller size I was when I married my husband. I went through bouts of depression about my size and was just pretty much a robot during intercourse (which is not me at all!). I wanted it completely dark so he couldn't see me.

My husband reassured me that he loved me no matter what size. However, I had to pray and dig real deep and realize that I am a sexy plus-size woman. Sexiness is a mindset and a self-confidence. But, I was determined to lose weight (not for my husband but for me). I desired to look better and to feel better.

Also, you will feel more romantic and sexual if you and your husband go "on a date" at least once a week, or once a month at a minimum. I know that may be too much for couples with small children; in such cases, just start out with once a month. "A date" does not mean money. Go for a ride together. Go for a long walk together. Put the kids in bed and have a picnic in your living room. Arrange with a loving couple with children to take care of their children for a few hours per month in exchange for them taking care of your children.

YOU NEED A DATE WITH YOUR HUSBAND; alone—no children and not with other couples. There's a time to go out with other couples. That is very valuable. However, you and your husband need to cultivate your own friendship and intimacy with each other apart from your children and friends.

I know couples that only talk together about their children. They have nothing else to talk about! Wives and husbands need hobbies together. Of course, he needs his own time and/or time with the "boys." Just like wives need their own time and/or time with "the girls." However, cultivate a hobby together. Play golf together. Play tennis together. Go bicycling together. Go for walks together.

Also ladies, spend quality time with your hubbies in the evening. If he wants you to watch television with him, sit with him for an hour. Forget about the laundry for that hour.

Ladies, your husbands want you to enjoy sex with them. They want you to "want him" and be vocal during sexual intercourse. During intercourse, he wants to hear your excitement, do not just lay there. Wives, if you are having sex with your husbands out of obligation your marriage will not be very satisfying to you nor him. Remember ladies; sex is God's idea. It is not just for procreation but also for building a stronger, healthier, happy marriage. So, enjoy!

Remember that sex is one of God's good gifts. God's intent is for sexual union to be expressed solely within the exclusive monogamous relationship of marriage. Human sexuality and sexual union within marriage were part of God's good design.